SELF-NEGLECT

A PRACTICAL APPROACH TO RISKS AND STRENGTHS ASSESSMENT

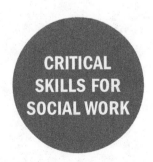

CRITICAL
SKILLS FOR
SOCIAL WORK

SELF-NEGLECT

A PRACTICAL APPROACH TO RISKS AND STRENGTHS ASSESSMENT

Shona Britten and Karen Whitby

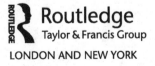

Routledge
Taylor & Francis Group

LONDON AND NEW YORK

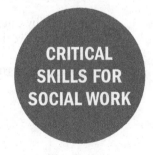

CRITICAL
SKILLS FOR
SOCIAL WORK

First published in 2018 by Critical Publishing Ltd

Published 2025 by Routledge
4 Park Square, Milton Park, Abingdon, Oxon OX14 4RN
605 Third Avenue, New York, NY 10017

Routledge is an imprint of the Taylor & Francis Group, an informa business

Copyright © 2018 Shona Britten and Karen Whitby

British Library Cataloguing in Publication Data
A CIP record for this book is available from the British Library

ISBN: 9781912096862 (pbk)
ISBN: 9781041056829 (ebk)

The rights of Shona Britten and Karen Whitby to be identified as the
Author of this work have been asserted by them in accordance
with the Copyright, Design and Patents Act 1988.

Cover design by Out of House
Text design by Greensplash Limited

DOI: 10.4324/9781041056829

Contents

Acknowledgements

We would like to express our sincere thanks in particular to Dr Mary Rose Day (DN, MA, PGDipPHN, BSc, RPHN, RM, RGN, Nurse Consultant, Co. Cork, Ireland; Part-time Lecturer at School of Nursing and Midwifery, University College Cork, Ireland) for her insight, support, and vast knowledge, generously shared with us from the point at which we first put 'our toes in the water' of authorship. This propelled us through to the publication of this book. Also we recognise and thank Dr Andrew Heighton (MBChB, MRCPsych) for his contributions to the development and consolidation of our thoughts in regard to this ever-evolving and multi-faceted area of practice.

We would also like to thank Mike Briggs (DSSM, DASS, CQSW), the national Adult Safeguarding co-lead for the Association of Directors of Adult Social Services (ADASS), for the interest he has expressed in our work. This was both motivating and reassuring to us, and added impetus to progress this work to publication.

Finally, we would like to share our absolute gratitude to Di Page for her warmth and guidance throughout our work with Critical Publishing, and of course to our families for their understanding, tolerance and humour.

Meet the authors

Shona began her career in social care in 1985, working for a charity supporting the carers of young adults with learning disabilities. As a qualified social worker Shona has worked with adults at risk, in both statutory and independent sector settings, holding a range of posts including multi-disciplinary team and area operational management; service planning and development in the areas of social inclusion and community development; and as a regional director. Shona continues to be directly engaged in social work practice on a consultancy basis and is registered with the HCPC.

Karen is a qualified and HCPC-registered social worker who has worked within the arena of health and social care for over 25 years. Karen's career in social care has involved managing learning disabilities and Carers and Safeguarding Adults services. She currently works as a lead professional for Safeguarding Adults within the NHS.

Foreword

I am pleased to welcome this timely book. Safeguarding adults is universally recognised as a prime task for all who are engaged in social and health care services or who deal with people who may be at risk of harm such as the Police or Housing. It is pleasing to see that self-neglect has now gained recognition as one of the conditions where people can be particularly at risk. This book offers an overview of the causes and effects of self-neglect, practical methods for dealing with the problem and rounds up the relevant legislation that is available to manage it.

Adult safeguarding has come a long way over the past 20 years to a point where it is now on a par with child safeguarding. The Care Act 2014 and subsequent government guidance has now established, within a legal framework, the roles and duties of organisations and their staff to work together to prevent adult abuse and to swiftly tackle it when it happens. In doing so the categorisation of adult safeguarding has been broadened to encompass self-neglect along with other associated areas such as domestic violence and modern-day slavery. As a result of improvements in safeguarding policy and practice there is more awareness among the general public, as evidenced by a growing rate of abuse and neglect referrals. This increase in demand, coupled with standstill or reduced budgets, means public sector services have had to refine their resources and staff training to ensure they prioritise referrals, comply with the new legislation and maximise their impact when they do intervene.

While organisations have moved to update their procedures and systems in response to increased responsibilities, there have been similar developments in the world of practice. A growing body of Safeguarding Adult Reviews has highlighted the need for good communication and a fully coordinated approach between all the workers who are involved with a person or their family. The concept of personalisation has been developed to form a new approach called Making Safeguarding Personal, which has been embraced by social workers and increasingly by Health Services and other key organisations. Through this approach people are no longer processed as a bystander but are placed at the centre of intervention and care planning – they are asked what outcomes they want and worked with as a partner in reaching the most desirable solution that makes them feel safer (where the person does not have the capacity to say what they want, then they are supported by an advocate).

Experience has told us that dealing effectively with someone who self-neglects is a joint enterprise. Safeguarding Adults boards have a duty to bring all the relevant organisations together to ensure they are working in partnership to make people safer, and many have focused on the issue of self-neglect through development sessions or audits. There is not a single solution but it is an area where some workers are better placed to intervene than others depending on individual and environmental factors. For example, Fire Services are often the only 'professional' that a reclusive person will let through their door; as well as using their expert knowledge they can also act as a bridge to social and health workers.

Self-neglect is one of those subjects that often gets filed in the 'too difficult to do' drawer when it involves someone who is clearly not coping but has mental capacity and a fierce independence that declines all offers of help. Such cases raise all sorts of quandaries such as 'what if they burn the house down? What if they fall and are left undiscovered? Should I take legal action to intervene?' The authors come at self-neglect from all angles, drawing on the knowledge bases of social work, medicine, nursing, psychology and the law along with their own extensive experience. They tackle the tricky issues of risk-taking, confidentiality and non-compliance from a practice-based perspective, not only acknowledging the dilemmas that face workers but offering them templates and down-to-earth advice. The strands of person-centred and coordinated approaches are threaded throughout the writing. The decision-making charts will help both practitioners and their managers, and the risk analysis tools will focus minds on how and when to intervene. Concise summaries of relevant legislation provide a tool chest from which to explore all the available statutory options. The result is an accessible guide for workers in the adult-safeguarding field and anyone who has the potential to come across someone who is self-neglecting. It should appeal to those who are already dealing with self-neglect but want to know more, or those wishing to update their knowledge of the latest developments.

Mike Briggs

Mike is currently the national Adult Safeguarding co-lead for the Association of Directors of Adult Social Services (ADASS); the independent chair of East Riding of Yorkshire Safeguarding Adults Board; chair of North East Lincolnshire Social Work Practice Community Interest Company's Board of Governors; an Associate of and lead peer reviewer for the Local Government Association (LGA); and advised on the drafting and subsequent guidance to safeguarding aspects of the Care Act (2014). He has worked on a range of developmental commissions for Councils and other public bodies; among other publications, he wrote the ADASS/LGA Safeguarding Advice and Guidance for Directors of Adult Social Services.

Person-centred care with people who self-neglect: from principles to practice

Over recent years the world of social care, particularly in relation to work with adults, has changed dramatically. These changes have seen a shift from a focus upon social workers as the commissioners of packages of care, to more full re-engagement with the professional values of empowerment, autonomy, and person-centred control. Social workers are viewed as enabling and supportive agents of change, with interventions centred upon the achievement of the priorities and outcomes that people themselves identify and want to achieve.

The Care Act (2014) has embedded 'person-centred' practice in primary legislation, supported by guidance which has statutory status. This climate of change has posed many challenges for all involved in the world of Adult Services to enable the translation of principles into effective operational practice. Not least is the understanding of neglect and self-neglect in terms of adult social care interventions, including safeguarding. The initial moves encapsulated within the Making Safeguarding Personal (MSP) agenda placed the need to embed person-centred practice at the forefront of all interventions in order to achieve positive and inclusive Safeguarding Adults work. This focus has also raised complex questions surrounding the interfaces and interrelationships of a person-centred practice approach with people who self-neglect and the Mental Capacity Act (2005) and Human Rights Act (1998).

Why we have written this book

This significant agenda for change prompted us, as practitioners, to look for some straightforward solutions to common-practice questions surrounding the need to respond appropriately to the increasing numbers of adults who self-neglect, or are at risk of self-neglecting, who come to the attention of Adult Services and partner agencies, commonly from concerns raised via Safeguarding Adults. This debate and search for solutions resulted in the development, for us, of a shared belief that practice-focused guidance was needed. Our thoughts have become this text, which is absolutely designed to be both meaningful and useful to practitioners

We have primarily aimed to describe a practical intervention framework and guide for a risks and strengths assessment approach in self-neglect, which supports staff who are working with adults who self-neglect, or may be at risk of self-neglecting in the future. This framework aims to offer:

> » a multi-agency resource in relation to self-neglect as a spectrum of factors or constellation of themes and complexity;
>
> » practice supports for preventive, early intervention and complex case work;
>
> » illustrative scenario examples which inform and support practitioners;
>
> » a risks and strengths assessment model supported by concise practice guidance *SnapShots* which contextualise factors in self-neglect and support structured interventions.

As experienced social-work practitioners, we have designed concise practical guides to key issues and concepts in self-neglect. These we have called *SnapShots*, and have found them to be of assistance to ourselves and colleagues. The *SnapShot* format is incorporated within the text in order to prompt and focus professional discussion, ongoing development and potentially initiate further research in this multi-faceted and growing area of work which is of concern both nationally and internationally. Each chapter concludes with *Taking it Further*; this element includes references and information resources which the reader may wish to explore in order to expand their knowledge and understanding of self-neglect.

How this book is structured

The style of this text is very much based upon meeting the practical day-to-day needs of professionals working with people who self-neglect, or are at risk of self-neglect. It can be used as an accessible resource to 'dip into' rather than as a piece of writing to be read from beginning to end. Each of the chapters, *SnapShots* and appendices can be used as standalone resources, as well as components of the comprehensive intervention framework and risks and strengths assessment model.

A brief overview of the content of each Chapter is given below in order to ease the reader's navigation of the text:

> **Chapter One** discusses the concept and contextual issues associated with self-neglect and factors for multi-agency consideration. *SnapShots* included are:
>
> > » clutter and extreme hoarding
> >
> > » Diogenes and Noah Syndromes
>
> **Chapter Two** details a practical model intervention framework for use in self-neglect cases, with illustrative examples and sample document formats. This suggested model is supported by full guidance notes and a set of *SnapShots*; these are:
>
> > » decision-making and disengagement

- » information-sharing
- » equality and diversity
- » fluctuating capacity
- » Lasting Power of Attorney (LPA)
- » independent advocacy
- » co-production
- » advance support planning

Chapter Three contains a risks and strengths assessment model, supported by full guidance notes, illustrative examples and sample document formats, including *SnapShots* which summarise:

- » driving and restraining forces to consider when utilising a conceptual risk assessment model – a human perspective
- » criminal offences and safeguarding adults
- » domestic abuse
- » The Modern Slavery Act (2015)
- » exploitation and illegal drug use
- » grooming
- » mate crime

Chapter Four looks at illustrative case scenarios using the risks and strengths assessment model framework and associated example documentation. A descriptive 'volcano effect' graphic is included as a visual learning tool.

Chapter Five considers the Care Act (2014) 'well-being' principle in self-neglect and Safeguarding Adults work. The *SnapShots* included in this chapter are:

- » balancing attitudes and values in person-centred safeguarding
- » The Care Act (2014) and supporting carers
- » a person in a position of trust

Chapter Six suggests an approach, developed by the authors, to building sustainable community strength and resilience. This model directly relates to and interfaces with the role of agencies represented on locality Safeguarding Adults Boards, in addressing self-neglect and the people who are at risk of self-neglect living in their area. The *SnapShot* in this chapter describes a suggested personalised community consolidation model of practice which places the person at the centre of all interventions from the individual through to multi-agency planning and decision-making.

The three appendices we have included with this work are:

1. A *SnapShot* Guide to the Mental Capacity Act (2005)

2. A *SnapShot* Guide to the Mental Health Act (1983) – rights, powers and protection

3. A *SnapShot* Guide to terminology in Safeguarding Adults

Our aim will have been met if practitioners find the content and format of our work informative and most importantly useful, as well as if it supports multi-agency planning and practice to converge in consistently achieving positive outcomes with adults at risk.

Introduction

This chapter discusses the concept and context of issues associated with people who self-neglect. It includes:

» examples of behaviours we have identified through our work with adults of all ages who self-neglect and are those which practitioners may come across in their work;

» what the *Care and Support Statutory Guidance* says about responses to self-neglect;

» multi-agency considerations in this complex area of work;

» a table outlining five Safeguarding Adults Reviews where self-neglecting behaviours were a factor;

» *SnapShots* on:

  » clutter and extreme hoarding;

  » Diogenes and Noah Syndromes.

What the the Care Act (2014) says about self-neglect

There are many varying complexities associated with the concept of 'self-neglect'; these have been recognised in both national and international research on the subject and are defined as priorities for action within the Care Act (2014); paragraph 14.17 of the Statutory Guidance states:

Self-neglect may not prompt a section 42 enquiry. An assessment should be made on a case by case basis. A decision on whether a response is required under safeguarding will depend on the adult's ability to protect themselves by controlling their own behaviour. There may come a point when they are no longer able to do this, without external support.

Factors associated with self-neglect in adults from practice

There are many presenting factors and behaviours which may, in varying combination, be indicative of self-neglect in adults. This wide range of factors can include, but are not limited to, the following examples:

» The failure of an individual to manage their physical and/or mental health, eg not taking medicines as prescribed; not seeking medical assistance and/or examination when needed; inadequate food, water and/or clothing; inadequate personal safety.

» Their involvement with individuals or groups which cause them harm, from which the individual is unable to withdraw, eg financial exploitation, physical assault.

» Unstable and inadequate housing, eg 'sofa-surfing', the threat of eviction from a rented property, living in a privately owned property which is unsafe.

» Environmental hazards within their home environment, eg problematic hoarding of objects and/or animals, lack of basic utilities, squalor.

» Social isolation and exclusion.

» Impaired cognition and/or physical disabilities, eg learning difficulties, mental health condition (including dementia-type conditions).

» Lack of insight or will to undertake essential daily hygiene/care tasks; the individual *may or may not* have mental capacity as defined within the requirements of the Mental Capacity Act (2005) Chapter Two, or they may experience fluctuations in their capacity to make a specific decision at the time the decision needs to be made. Fluctuations in mental capacity may be severely influenced by the abuse of alcohol or drugs, or prescribed medicines.

NB: This is not an exhaustive list.

Multi-agency considerations

Despite the acceptance of self-neglect as a matter of concern for the individuals themselves, agencies and the wider public, difficulties in achieving positive outcomes for the person concerned remain; this can be due in part to some of the points identified below:

» Those supporting the person who is self-neglecting are often unaware of which other agencies can offer input, support and advice.

» Some organisations and agencies have not prioritised or given consideration to the long-term issues of self-neglect and historically have not engaged fully with multi-agency responses.

» People can 'fall through the gap' of services, and their situations can deteriorate to a catastrophic level without input.

» The allocation of resources between organisations and agencies may often not be effectively coordinated.

Self-neglect is complex and multi-faceted; it can cover areas of responsibility held by all local statutory agencies including the Police Authority; Fire and Rescue Services; Environmental Health Departments; NHS Trusts; Clinical Commissioning Groups; Adult Social Care; Housing Departments; Probation Services; Multi-agency Public Protection Arrangements (MAPPA); Multi-agency Risk Assessment Conferences (MARAC); RSPCA; Children and Families Social Care; as well as Safeguarding Adults Boards and Safeguarding Children Boards.

Due to the diversity in presentation of self-neglect this can lead to devastating and catastrophic outcomes for the individual, when not recognised and addressed by the organisations and agencies involved. In these cases the organisations and agencies can find themselves placed in vulnerable and potentially serious situations in safeguarding due to a lack of clear understanding regarding:

» the extent to which self-neglect is prevalent in their areas of responsibility;

» the nature of self-neglecting behaviours and their impact upon the health, well-being and safety of the individual themselves and others, both current and in the future;

» priorities for service developments and commissioning to meet the future need.

Safeguarding Adults Reviews (SARs)

Safeguarding Adults Boards (SABs) have a statutory duty under the Care Act (2014) Section 44 to arrange for a Safeguarding Adults Review (SAR) to be undertaken in particular circumstances. The *Care and Support Statutory Guidance* (paragraphs 14.162–63) confirms the circumstances in which a SAR should be undertaken:

» *SABs must arrange a SAR when an adult in its area dies as a result of abuse or neglect, whether known or suspected, and there is concern that partner agencies could have worked more effectively to protect the adult;*

» *SABs must also arrange a SAR if an adult in its area has not died, but the SAB knows or suspects that the adult has experienced serious abuse or neglect. In the context of SARs, something can be considered serious abuse or neglect where, for example the individual would have been likely to have died but for an intervention, or has suffered permanent harm or has reduced capacity or quality of life (whether because of physical or psychological effects) as a result of the abuse or neglect. SABs are free to arrange for a SAR in any other situations involving an adult in its area with needs for care and support.*

The records of cases which have sadly led to the death of an adult, for whom self-neglect was a factor in their life, included within published SARs and those reports previously known as Serious Case Reviews (SCRs), can provide vital resources of 'lessons learned' and action plans implemented; examples are contained below in Table 1.1. The translation of 'lessons learned' into core operational procedure remains an area for ongoing development, which requires the membership of SABs to achieve clarity regarding the prevalence rates in their own area in order to support local and national service design and commissioning priorities; this relationship is described by the authors as Personalised Community Consolidation and is discussed in Chapter 6.

Table 1.1 Safeguarding Adult Review examples

Case	Overview Context	Reference
Deceased female adult (43 years of age). Cause of death: liver failure; alcohol cirrhosis; renal failure; septicaemia; infected fracture. Author's note: Potential for fluctuations in mental capacity while under the influence of alcohol (not documented within available report).	History of alcohol abuse. Insanitary living conditions: 'Police found the house to be in a very poor state with faeces and urine on the floor.' Reluctance to accept support. History of domestic violence. Mental health assessment concluded no severe or enduring mental illness. Previous CVA – aged 39 years (approx.), resulted in speech difficulties.	Serious Case Review regarding X. Cornwall Safeguarding Adults Board 2008
Deceased male adult. Cause of death: pneumonia; paranoid schizophrenia; inanition (starvation). Date of death: not known; pronounced dead: 25/03/2009 (found in his home). Mental capacity was assumed.	Misuse of prescribed and 'over-the-counter' medicines. Poor physical health; 'pressure sores'; concerns regarding the home environment – signs of self-neglecting behaviours. Depression; anxiety; behavioural problems; paranoid schizophrenia (partial lobotomy surgery); gastric problems.	Serious Case Review relating to A1. Worcestershire Safeguarding Adults Board April 2010
Deceased male adult (42 years of age). In line with Mental Capacity Act (2005) principles Mr AA was presumed to hold mental capacity.	Self-neglect of personal hygiene, diet and home environment. Lack of availability of prescribed medicine. Schizophrenia.	Safeguarding Adults Review Mr AA. Norfolk Safeguarding Adults Board June 2015

Case	Overview Context	Reference
Deceased male adult (under 65 years of age). Cause of death: 'sudden unexpected death in alcohol and peripheral vascular disease'. The Coroner confirmed 'that Mr I had been dead for some days.' Assessed to hold mental capacity to decide where and how he lived his life. Author's note: Potential for fluctuations in mental capacity while under the influence of alcohol.	Refusal to accept commissioned care and support services to meet essential personal health and social care needs. Ongoing involvement from local health and social care professionals. Self-neglect of personal health, prescribed medicines, diet and home environment to insanitary levels. Brain injury; lower leg amputation. History of depression. Severe dependence on alcohol.	Safeguarding Adults Review Mr I. West Berkshire Safeguarding Adults Board July 2016
Deceased female adult (34 years). The Coroner recorded an open verdict as the cause of death could not be ascertained. Ms T was found dead at her home; her body was in an advanced state of decomposition.	The SAR raised several issues, included were the following two practice points: 1. The difficulty that staff encountered around how best to act when the person at the centre of the concerns is not willing to accept help, or at best, to do so on his/her own terms. 2. The fact that this was a case of self-neglect and this may have affected the way in which Safeguarding functioned as there was no 'perpetrator'. Ms T had mental health problems, a history of asthma and type 2 diabetes which was not managed effectively.	Safeguarding Adults Review Ms T. Buckinghamshire Safeguarding Adults Board August 2017

It is vital to identify the nature of self-neglect, as well as the extent and impact of it on a case-by-case basis, as the support and/or intervention which may be required is unique to the person at the centre of the situation. It is recognised that there are people who present self-neglecting behaviours who, even with ongoing involvement and intervention, will not cooperate and engage with support planning. In these circumstances it is for the Lead Agency involved to consider statutory duties and responsibilities in line with current legislation; a brief overview of applicable legislation at the time of writing is given below in the *SnapShot on …* clutter and extreme hoarding (this is not exhaustive, and is not designed to provide any form of legal guidance).

Practice experience has, with retrospective review, supported the authors to promote the use of a clear and concise risks and strengths model of assessment by practitioners across all applicable agencies. This model of intervention addresses the serious concerns of self-neglect from a person-centered perspective and is described in detail in Chapters 2 and 3.

Practice matters ...

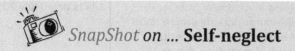

SnapShot on ... **Self-neglect**

Key issues to consider with adults of all ages who self-neglect are:

» Abuse, exploitation and criminal activity, which may also involve and/or impact upon children or other adults at risk who also reside within the property.

» Historical information in relation to childhood neglect and disordered attachment.

» Robust and consistent Risk Assessment, which identifies *hazards*, balanced with *strengths*, required/agreed *actions* focused upon the individual's views of their needs, and their ability to undertake and complete identified tasks.

» The need for Advocacy.

» Other agencies which can offer input, support and advice.

» The longer-term issues of self-neglect and multi-agency involvement.

» People who have or are at risk of 'falling through the gap' of services; it is known that these types of situation can deteriorate to a catastrophic level without input.

» The effective coordination and allocation of resources between organisations and agencies.

SnapShot on ... **Clutter and extreme hoarding**

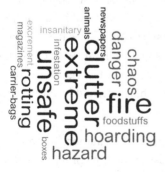

Clutter and extreme hoarding are facets of the broader issue of self-neglect. A simple definition of this is one of the refusal or impotence of an individual to safely manage and maintain their personal health, safety and well-being; this may be characterised in many ways including the maintenance of a safe living environment.

The classic presentation of clutter and extreme hoarding includes the hazardous accumulation of items which have no continuing use, and are NOT part of an ongoing or previous interest; such items can include old foodstuffs, packaging, newspapers, magazines and circulars as well as excrement. These behaviours can include the hoarding of animals in an unmanaged and chaotic manner; this is further discussed within the *SnapShot on ...* Diogenes and Noah syndromes below.

This type of self-neglecting behaviour and presentation can and does pose challenges for those involved with a person living in these circumstances as they may either refuse or be impotent to address the safety issues raised. People who hoard may have an acute association with their possessions, and refuse to regard them as hazardous and problematic to themselves and/or others. This pattern of extreme behaviour can be of significant detriment to the health and well-being of the occupant(s) of the property and potentially their neighbours. These risks can include infestation by rodents and insects, as well as fire risk and animal safety.

This situation requires a steady, dedicated and coordinated multi-agency approach with the involvement of potentially a range of statutory agencies in order to achieve safe and sustainable solutions. The accurate assessment of the individual's mental capacity is critical in these circumstances. In relation to the hoarding of animals, applicable animal safety agencies should be contacted immediately.

The completion of consistent and person-centred risk assessment, with the individual concerned, should recognise their strengths and personal solutions to the situation alongside legal responsibilities, which in England and Wales currently includes (in brief):

» The Care Act (2014)

» Mental Capacity Act (2005)

» Mental Health Act (1983)

» Human Rights Act (1989)

» Animal Welfare Act (2006)

» Environmental Protection Act (1990)

» Public Health Act (1936)

» Police and Criminal Evidence Act (1984)

» Gas Act (1986) and Electricity Act (1989)

» Housing Act (2004)

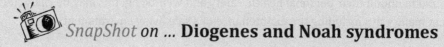

SnapShot on ... **Diogenes and Noah syndromes**

Rejection Contamination Isolation Animals Infestation Extreme Hoarding Infirmity Self-Neglect Unhealthiness Squalor

Diogenes syndrome was included within the 'Diagnostic and Statistical Manual of Mental Disorders', 5th Edition (DSM-5; *American Psychiatric Association*, 2013) as a behavioural condition which is typified by self-neglect, extreme hoarding, and environmental squalor; it is commonly associated and prevalent within the older adult population who reject available support and appear to lack insight into the risks and hazards.

Diogenes syndrome is named after the ancient Greek philosopher Diogenes of Sinope, who lived circa 412–323 BC. Diogenes was a contemporary of Plato, and is reported to have frequently challenged Plato's philosophical thinking and teachings. Contrary to the factors which are used to identify or diagnose Diogenes syndrome, it is reported that the man himself rejected all material possessions and lived, at times, in a large barrel.

Noah syndrome is described as a form of Diogenes syndrome in an article by Alejandra Saldarriaga-Cantillo MD and Juan Carlos Rivas MD. This research paper notes that in addition to the characteristics recognised as features in Diogenes syndrome the person affected will also hoard a *'large number of animals, neglecting their basic care and showing an inability to recognize the consequences this may have for the health and well-being of both the animals and the patient themselves.'* (Saldarriaga-Cantillo and Rivas, 2015, pp 1–2).

The acquisition of animals may occur passively, in that the person may have them given to them to be cared for or alternatively they may actively seek them out; in both cases the risk of uncontrolled reproduction is a key factor.

This syndrome may in part be so called in reference to Genesis Chapter 6: 19/20, where the instructions given to Noah included:

> *You are to bring into the ark two of all living creatures, male and female, to keep them alive with you.*

> *Two of every kind of bird, of every kind of animal and of every kind of creature that moves along the ground will come to you to be kept alive.*

and Genesis Chapter 7: 2/3:

> *Take with you seven pairs of every kind of clean animal, a male and its mate, and one pair of every kind of unclean animal, a male and its mate,*

> *and also seven pairs of every kind of bird, male and female, to keep their various kinds alive throughout the earth.*

In summary, this chapter has aimed to describe the multi-faceted nature of self-neglect and the need for a case by case approach to be taken by practitioners in the evaluation and planning of practice interventions with the person at the centre of all activities. Its purpose has also been to inform, prompt and focus further ongoing work for SABs and their partner agencies to engage fully with understanding the risks associated with self-neglect to ensure that service design and commissioning meets their community's priorities.

Taking it Further

Publications

Biswas, G, Bala, N and Choudhary, S (2013) Diogenes Syndrome: A Case Report. *Case Reports in Dermatological Medicine*.

Braye, S, Orr, D and Preston-Shoot, M (2011) Conceptualising and Responding to Self-Neglect: Challenges for Adult Safeguarding. *Journal of Adult Protection*, 13(4): 182–93.

Braye, S, Preston-Shoot, M and Orr, D (2012) The Governance of Adult Safeguarding: Findings from Research. *Journal of Adult Protection*, 14(2): 55–72.

Braye, S, Orr, D and Preston-Shoot, M (2015) Learning Lessons about Self-Neglect? An Analysis of Serious Case Reviews. *Journal of Adult Protection*, 17(1): 3–18.

Braye, S, Orr, D and Preston-Shoot, M (2015) Serious Case Review Findings on the challenges of self-Neglect: Indicators for Good Practice. *Journal of Adult Protection*, 17(2): 75–87.

Briggs, M (2013) *Safeguarding Adults: Advice and Guidance to Directors of Adult Social Services*. ADASS/LGA.

Burnett, J, Achenbaum, W A, Hayes, L, Flores, D V, Hochschild, A E, Kao, D, Halphen, J M and Dyer, C B (2012) Increasing Surveillance and Prevention Efforts for Elder Self-Neglect in Clinical Settings. *Aging Health*, 8(6): 647–55.

Day, M R and McCarthy, G (2016) Animal Hoarding: A Serious Public Health Issue. *Annals of Nursing and Practice*, 3(4): 1054.

Day, M R and McCarthy, G (2016) Self-neglect: Development and Evaluation of a Self-Neglect (SN-37) Measurement Instrument. *Archives of Psychiatric Nursing*, 30: 480–85.

Day, M R, Mulcahy, H, Leahy-Warren, P and Downey, J (2015) Self-neglect: A Case Study and Implications for Clinical Practice. *British Journal of Community Nursing*, 20(3): 110–14.

Iris, M, Ridings, J W and Conrad, K J (2010) The Development of a Conceptual Model for Understanding Elder Self-neglect. *The Gerontologist*, 50(3): 303–15.

Iris, M, Conrad, K J and Ridings, J (2014) Observational Measure of Elder Self-Neglect. *Journal of Elder Abuse & Neglect*, 26: 365–97.

Irvine, J and Nwachukwu, K (2014) Recognizing Diogenes Syndrome: A Case Report. *BMC Research Notes*, 7: 276.

Lauder, W, Roxburgh, M, Harris, J and Law, J (2009) Developing Self-Neglect Theory: Analysis of Related and Atypical Cases of People Identified as Self-Neglecting. *Journal of Psychiatric and Mental Health Nursing*, 16: 447–54.

Preston-Shoot, M (2016) Towards Explanations for the Findings of Serious Case Reviews: Understanding What Happens in Self-neglect Work. *Journal of Adult Protection*, 18(3): 131–48.

Williams, H, Clarke, R, Fashola, Y and Holt, G (1998) Diogenes' Syndrome in Patients with Intellectual Disability: 'A Rose By Any Other Name'? *Journal of Intellectual Disability Research*, 42: 316–20.

References

American Psychiatric Association (2013) *Diagnostic and Statistical Manual of Mental Disorders* (5th edn). Washington, DC: American Psychiatric Publishing.

Buckinghamshire Safeguarding Adults Board (2017) Safeguarding Adults Review Adult T Overview Report. [online] Available at: www.hampshiresab.org.uk/wp-content/uploads/Bucks-SAR-Case-T-Final.pdf (accessed 20 November 2017).

Cornwall Safeguarding Adults Board (formerly Cornwall Adult Protection Committee) (2008) Executive Summary of a Serious Case Review in Respect an Adult Female Who Died 12th March 2007. [online] Available at: www.hampshiresab.org.uk/wp-content/uploads/2008-Serious-Case-Review-regarding-X-Cornwall.pdf (accessed 16 May 2017).

Department of Health (2017) *The Care and Support Statutory Guidance*.

Norfolk Safeguarding Adults Board and Suffolk Safeguarding Adults Board (2015) Safeguarding Adult Review in respect of Mr AA Died January 2014. (11/11/2015). Available online at www.norfolksafeguardingadultsboard. info/safeguarding-adults-review/safeguarding-adult-review-mr-aa-published-november-2015 (accessed 16 May 2017).

Saldarriaga-Cantillo, A and Rivas, J C (2015) Noah Syndrome: A Variant of Diogenes Syndrome Accompanied by Animal Hoarding Practices. *Journal of Elder Abuse & Neglect*, 27(3): 270–5.

The Stationery Office on behalf of the Department for Constitutional Affairs (2007) *The Mental Capacity Act Code of Practice*.

West of Berkshire Safeguarding Adults Board (2016) Safeguarding Adult Review Mr I. [online] Available at: www. hampshiresab.org.uk/wp-content/uploads/SAR-Mr-I-Final-Report-2016v4.pdf (accessed 16 May 2017).

Worcestershire Safeguarding Adults Board (2010) Executive Summary April 2010 Serious Case Review Relating To A. [online] Available at: www.hampshiresab.org.uk/wp-content/uploads/2010-April-Serious-Case-Review-regarding-A1-Worcestershire.pdf (accessed 16 May 2017).

Introduction

In this chapter we introduce and describe a practical model intervention framework for use in self-neglect cases, which is supported by illustrative examples and sample document formats. This framework format has developed over our years of social work practice with adults of all ages and has supported us to take a structured approach in our work, which we have found to be both logical and most importantly supportive. We have strengthened our suggested model with simple guidance notes and a set of *SnapShots* which describe several important areas of practice.

>   » Decision-making and disengagement
>   » Information-sharing
>   » Equality and diversity
>   » Fluctuating mental capacity
>   » Lasting Power of Attorney (LPA)
>   » Independent advocacy
>   » Co-production
>   » Advance support planning

Our aim is to provide a positive approach to the complex and challenging practice issues which can be associated with working to engage people who self-neglect in care and support processes.

A model intervention framework

In itself this self-neglect intervention framework is not a solution to the issue of self-neglect but rather a means to support multi- or single-agency informed proactive practice and proposed lines of accountability. Its aim is multi-faceted, and focused upon:

>   » supporting effective practice for frontline staff;
>   » the creation of robust monitoring (needs analysis) and reporting mechanisms for responsible agencies;
>   » the promotion of clarity in decision-making processes;
>   » enabling cooperative, cost- and resource-effective multi-agency working;

and most importantly

> » the achievement of positive outcomes for the adult at the centre of the intervention and their family, carers and supporters who are willing to accept support.

The self-neglect intervention framework (Table 2.1) is designed to provide guidance for each element of the assessment and decision-making process from initial contact through to:

> » signposting *or* referral to applicable agencies/support services;

> » the agreement and implementation of a Safeguarding Support Plan;

> » consideration of the need to exercise applicable statutory/legislative responsibilities by the identified Lead Agency, including implementation of a Disengagement Policy/Procedure as applicable and appropriate.

As an aid to interpretation the following guidance is divided under section headings:

Section 1 – Initial information gathering

It is vital at this stage to gather as much applicable information as possible. This should include the following elements; however, it must be noted that this is not an exhaustive list, and existing agency formats should be followed with professional judgement:

> » historic information including contact with Children's Services, and any previous Safeguarding concerns;

> » known mental or physical health conditions;

> » details of the involvement with local agencies, eg Police, Housing, Environmental Health, Criminal Justice, etc;

> » housing tenure (private, rented);

> » homelessness (eg bed and breakfast accommodation, 'sofa-surfing', etc);

> » children and/or other adults residing at or regularly visiting the property;

> » animals kept at the property;

> » any communication needs and/or barriers;

> » the length of time concerns regarding self-neglect have been known.

Section 2 – Lead Agency identification

Following the gathering and analysis of information regarding the potential risk of self-neglect occurring, a decision should be made based upon these details of which agency is best placed to make enquiries and undertake a visit to the property. As an example, it may have become apparent that there has been a neighbour dispute which has involved the Housing Department; in this type of case they may be confirmed as the Lead Agency, or the Police may be involved in criminal investigations, in which case they would be the Lead Agency. This decision-making process must be recorded and clearly documented.

Section 3 and 4 – Risks and strengths assessment

The guidance notes which accompany the self-neglect risks and strengths assessment model (detailed in Chapter 3) must be followed in order to identify the level and grading of risk associated with an individual case. Severe problematic hoarding behaviours must be distinguished from an individual's choice to collect items, and acknowledgement given to the potential emotional attachment the adult at risk may have to such items.

A *MODERATE* or *LOW* grading may indicate that the individual should be encouraged and supported to engage with local support services, such as local cleaning services, etc. As emphasised above, professional judgement must be made in each individual case, as intervention may be required to militate against the risk of further deterioration.

A *HIGH* or *CRITICAL* grading would commonly indicate that immediate actions are required to safeguard the individual's health and safety. At this point multi-agency involvement should be sought, in order that:

1. the appropriate Lead Agency and Worker be confirmed;
2. an Action Plan be agreed

Throughout the risk assessment process, should it become apparent that there are concerns for the safety and/or welfare of children, other adults at risk, and/or animals within the property or associated with the individual, these must be reported to applicable agency(ies) within required timescales.

Section 5, 6 and 8 – Acceptance of support and advocacy

In cases of self-neglect it is quite common for individuals to refuse to cooperate with the intervention of others. This is a complex balance of legal human rights to lifestyle choice, through to Mental Capacity Act (2005) Assessment, assessment under the Mental Health Act (1983), public safety and criminal justice legislation. In cases where the individual accepts support, consideration should be given to the involvement of an independent advocate in order that they are supported to be actively involved in the co-production of an appropriate Action Plan.

Where an individual refuses to be involved or accept support, in line with legislative requirements noted above, there should be concerted efforts made to engage positively with them and any carers, family and/or friends. This process of seeking engagement can extend over prolonged periods of time and should be consistently and positively pursued. This element of cooperation and co-production of Support Plans is a vital element in seeking minimal risk of relapse. However, at times implementation of an agreed Disengagement Policy and Procedure may be required.

The involvement of an independent advocate may, over an extended period of time, act as a means to reassure and encourage the individual that support can and should be accepted as a positive decision.

Section 7 – Further consideration

Where an Action Plan has been implemented, and the individual continues to refuse to cooperate, further consideration should be given to any other underlying factors which may be preventing or inhibiting them. This may include, for example, the involvement of the individual's GP, Community Mental Health Services, the Police or Safeguarding Adults Officers.

All actions planned must be, as applicable, based upon:

» Mental Capacity Act (2005) Assessment and documented Best Interest Decision-making;

» Registered Lasting Power of Attorney (finance and/or welfare);

» Mental Health Act (1983) Assessment and/or Aftercare requirements;

» Environmental Health and/or Fire Safety Hazards;

» The Police and/or Probation Service involvement.

Section 9 – Multi-agency Safeguarding Support Plan

The Safeguarding Support Plan should be completed, agreed and implemented. This should be reviewed within the confirmed timescale, or sooner should circumstances change. This should also include applicable 'Contingency Plans' (illustrative examples are described in Chapter 4).

The self-neglect risks and strengths assessment model should be used to review the effect-iveness of the Safeguarding Support Plan, and as a means to evidence the management and/or reduction of applicable risk factors.

Section 10 – Disengagement and statutory duties

The multi-agency team should consider applicable legislation and refer to their legal department(s) for guidance as required. This may include the implementation of an agreed Disengagement Policy and Procedure.

This risks and strengths assessment model supports an evaluation to be made in respect of *key* social and healthcare factors which potentially impact upon the likelihood that an adult at risk will be at risk of harm and the impact(s) of those risks in line with organisational responsibilities.

Table 2.1 Intervention Framework

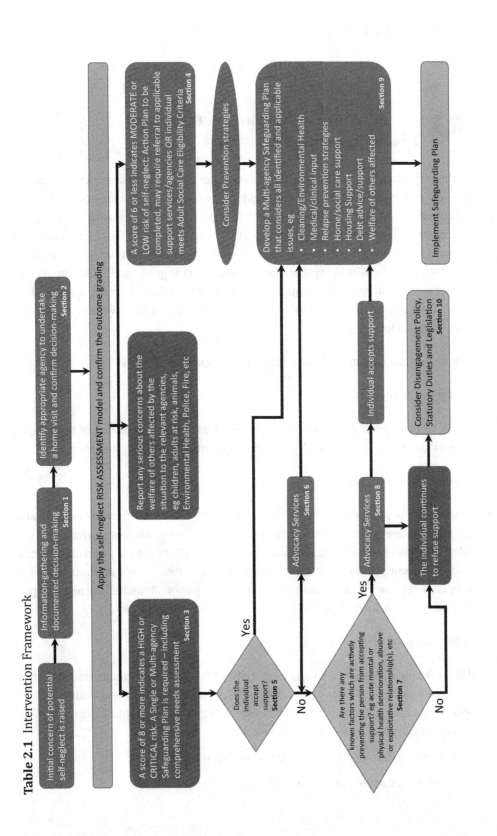

Practice matters ...

SnapShot on ... **Decision-making and disengagement**

In the majority of cases it is not problematic when a person chooses not to attend or engage with some or all of the services offered to them but there are occasions when this can give cause for concern. The findings of the National Confidential Enquiry into Suicide and Homicide by People with Mental Illness – Safer Services (1999) included a loss of contact with services as a frequent feature of suicide and homicide enquiries. It is 'best practice' within organisations to have specific guidance in relation to cases of disengagement and non-compliance, which gives staff a structure within which they can maximise the efficiency of their efforts to support those who do not engage well with services.

Simple working definitions of 'disengagement and non-compliance'

a) Difficult to engage:

There is a history of disengagement with services and sufficient risk of harm being caused to self and/or others which negates the option of closing the case.

b) Non-compliance/non-engagement:

The words *compliance* and *engagement* should not obscure the fact that unless statutory powers are in place, a person has the *right* to refuse treatment and/or services – what constitutes non-compliance and/or non-engagement will vary on a case-by-case basis. For example, the significance and meaning of two missed appointments will vary greatly between one person and another – no policy eliminates the need for professional judgement, evaluation and assessment of associated risk(s).

c) Non-attendance:

This is frequently referred to and recorded as DNA (Did Not Attend), and is used to describe a person who has been referred to, or has an appointment with, a service, and fails to attend at the agreed time, date or venue. For example, a person may be classed as DNA in the following circumstances:

» the person does not attend the initial assessment interview;

» the person does not attend an outpatient or therapy session;

» the person is not at home when visited at a previously agreed/confirmed date and time;

» the person does not attend a regular activity on one or more occasions (in some cases a single occasion will raise concern, and action is required);

» the person has moved from their usual place of residence and given no forwarding address.

Examples of potential reasons for 'disengagement and non-compliance':

» Lack of accessible and meaningful information regarding the support being offered (for example, does the person use sign language, MAKATON, or do they require translation into their first language or another accessible format?).

» Poor relationship between the person and the provider of the care/support offered.

» Experience of adverse side-effects of treatment.

» Lack of insight and/or understanding of the benefits of the care, support, intervention offered.

Factors to consider in practice:

1. The RIGHT to refuse care/support:

    a. While every effort should be made to support the engagement of the person, it must be recognised that if they have the mental capacity (Mental Capacity Act (2005) Section 1 (2)) they have the right to refuse input even if this is considered to be an unwise choice/decision.

    b. However, based upon the individual case, consideration should be given to use of the Mental Health Act (1983); for example, detention, assessment, treatment, Guardianship, Community Treatment Order, Aftercare, etc.

    c. If the person lacks the mental capacity to make this decision (Mental Capacity Act (2005) Section 2 (1)), there is a legal requirement to act in their Best Interests in those areas where they are assessed to lack capacity to decide to refuse services; all actions should be proportionate to identified risk(s) and be clearly documented.

2. The terms 'disengaged' and 'non-compliant', when attached to a person, may carry a tone which infers that they are difficult. It is vitally important to remember to investigate the reasons for their refusal to engage – it may be that what is being offered is not helpful to them. Always have open discussions with the person about this, particularly in respect the potential reasons noted above.

3. Any and all professionals involved with a person who disengages or is non-compliant should inform the case co-ordinator as soon as possible (see Figure 2.1 below). The case co-ordinator should then identify and assess all relevant risk factors and plan accordingly, making use of information from all other agencies and individuals involved.

Figure 2.1 Decision-making in disengagement and non-compliance

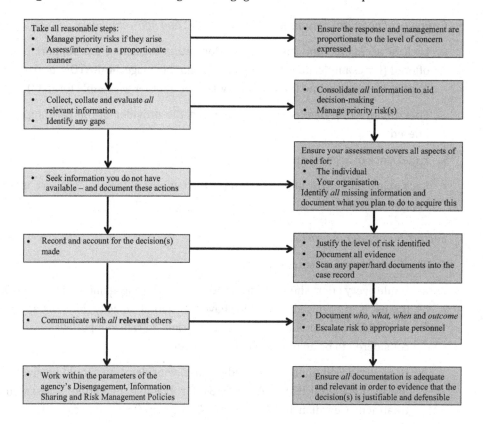

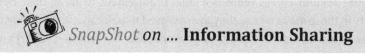 *SnapShot* on ... **Information Sharing**

In order to respond appropriately, where abuse or neglect may be taking place, anyone in contact with the adult, whether in a voluntary or paid role, must understand their own role and responsibilities. They should also have access to practical and legal guidance, advice and support. This will include understanding local inter-agency policies and procedures, such as the Safeguarding Adults Board (SAB), Multi-agency Policy and Procedure, Multi-Agency Risk Assessment Conference (MARAC) and Multi-agency Public Protection Arrangements (MAPPA).

» A MARAC is a meeting where information is shared on the highest-risk domestic abuse cases between representatives of local Police, health, child protection, housing practitioners, Independent Domestic Violence Advisors (IDVAs), probation and other specialists from the statutory and voluntary sectors.

» MAPPA are in place to ensure the successful management of violent and sexual offenders.

Your organisation's policies (or agreed ways of working) will give you guidance on safeguarding prevention and early intervention procedures to follow if and when abuse or neglect has happened or is suspected.

Where there are Safeguarding Adult concerns, staff have a duty to share information. It is important to remember that in a number of Safeguarding Adults Reviews (SARs, previously known as Serious Case Reviews) ineffective information-sharing has been identified as a prominent factor. For example, this is described as a factor within the Safeguarding Adults Review (SAR) undertaken by the West Berkshire Safeguarding Adults Board (SAB) published in July 2016 regarding an adult named Mr I. This SAR report highlights particular issues in relation to the completion of case transfer processes, which took place during and following a period of agency restructure and included the updating of and access to key electronic care records across service disciplines; in this case a Single Point of Access function and mental health services.

Staff should have clear direction in what information should be recorded and in what format. A key consideration for any individual involved with suspected or actual abuse or neglect should be 'What information am I required to share and with whom, in order to manage the risk?' (see Figure 2.2 below: The Critical Question Wheel)

Figure 2.2 The Critical Question Wheel

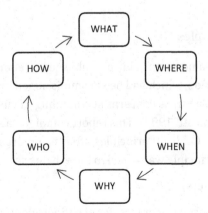

Seven *golden* rules in Adult Safeguarding

1. The Data Protection Act (1998) is not a barrier to the sharing of information, but provides a framework to ensure that the personal information of living persons is managed and shared appropriately (see Figure 2.3: Flowchart of key aspects in information-sharing).

2. Be open and honest with the person (and/or their family or representative as appropriate) from the onset about *why*, *what*, *how* and with *whom* information will or could be shared. Seek their agreement unless it is unsafe or inappropriate to do so (document all decisions, confirming how they were arrived at).

3. Seek advice if you are in doubt – without disclosing the identity of the person where possible.

4. Share information with the consent of the person where possible and appropriate – respect the wishes of those who do not give consent to the sharing of information, while remembering that you may still do so *if* in your judgement the lack of consent can be overridden in the public interest. Judgements must be based upon the facts of the case.

5. Consider *safety* and *well-being* – base your information-sharing decisions on consideration of the safety and well-being of the person and others who may be affected by their actions (eg carers).

6. *Necessary, proportionate, relevant, accurate, timely, secure*: ensure that the information you share is necessary for the purpose for which you are sharing it – these six factors are commonly referred to as the Caldicott principles (further information is detailed below).

7. Keep a clear chronological record of *all* decisions, and the reasons they were made.

The Caldicott principles

In December 1997, Dame Fiona Caldicott published a Report on the Review of Patient-identifiable Information, which had been commissioned in 1997 by the Chief Medical Officer in England to address concerns surrounding the use of personal information within the NHS (Caldicott, 1997). This report contained a set of six principles, which became known as the Caldicott principles, after the report's author. In 2012, following a review a seventh principle was added to the existing set. These seven principles are:

1. Justify the purpose(s).

   Every single proposed use or transfer of patient-identifiable information within or from an organisation should be clearly defined and scrutinised, with continuing uses regularly reviewed, by an appropriate guardian.

2. Don't use patient-identifiable information unless it is necessary.

    Patient-identifiable information items should not be included unless they are essential for the specified purpose(s) of that flow. The need for patients to be identified should be considered at each stage of satisfying the purpose(s).

3. Use the minimum necessary patient-identifiable information.

    Where use of patient-identifiable information is considered to be essential, the inclusion of each individual item of information should be considered and justified so that the minimum amount of identifiable information is transferred or accessible as is necessary for a given function to be carried out.

4. Access to patient-identifiable information should be on a strict need-to-know basis.

    Only those individuals who need access to patient-identifiable information should have access to it, and they should only have access to the information items that they need to see. This may mean introducing access controls or splitting information flows where one information flow is used for several purposes.

5. Everyone with access to patient-identifiable information should be aware of their responsibilities.

    Action should be taken to ensure that those handling patient-identifiable information – both clinical and non-clinical staff – are made fully aware of their responsibilities and obligations to respect patient confidentiality.

6. Understand and comply with the law.

    Every use of patient-identifiable information must be lawful. Someone in each organisation handling patient information should be responsible for ensuring that the organisation complies with legal requirements.

7. The duty to share information can be as important as the duty to protect patient confidentiality

    Professionals should in the patient's interest share information within this framework. Official policies should support them in doing so.

Figure 2.3 Flowchart of key aspects in information-sharing
(adapted from: Guidance for Practitioners & Managers, HM Gov., March 2009)

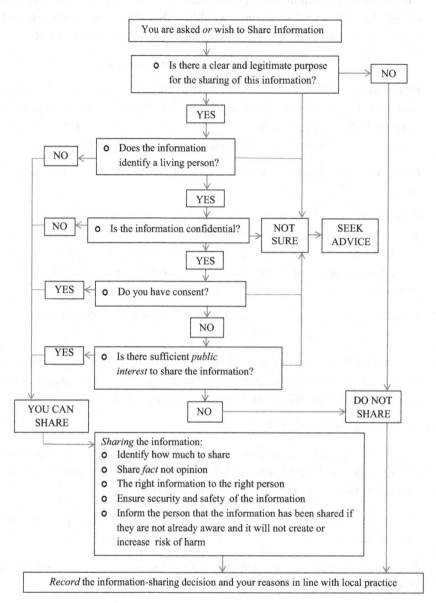

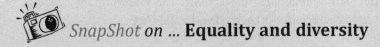

SnapShot on … **Equality and diversity**

An emphasis is placed upon the recognition that everyone is an individual with their own unique values, attitudes, beliefs and preferences. To achieve an approach to Safeguarding Adults that is 'person-centered', all of those involved need to recognise and respect individuality and diversity, while consulting with and involving the adult at risk at all stages of their journey through safeguarding.

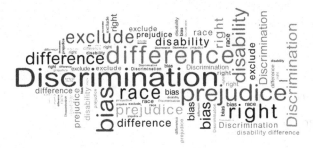

Equality and diversity are integral components in health and social care, as in practice we come into contact with some of the most complex, disadvantaged and marginalised groups within our communities. Practice which promotes equality and diversity ensures that those who are being supported are offered services which are fair and accessible to all. This is particularly important for adults at risk who are unable to take adequate care of themselves or to put appropriate strategies in place to safeguard themselves from abuse, neglect or harm.

Equality

Ensures that individuals or groups of individuals are not treated differently, or less favourably, on the basis of their specific identity.

Diversity

Aims to recognise, respect and value characteristic differences in people, and to pro-actively support an inclusive culture within society which promotes contributions from all to realise the achievement of full potential.

What the law says about equality and diversity

The Equalities Act (2010) replaced previous anti-discrimination legislation in order to establish a single piece of legislation within a simpler framework which removed inconsistencies and strengthened protections. The following are headings of the specific protected characteristics covered within this Act:

Protected characteristics relate to:

» Age

» Disability

» Gender reassignment

» Race

» Religion or belief

» Sex

» Sexual orientation

» Marriage and civil partnership

» Pregnancy and maternity

Unlawful treatment

Under the Equalities Act (2010), people whose identity is included within the nine protected characteristics confirmed above cannot lawfully be treated unfairly. The Act defines treatment considered to be unlawful as:

Direct Discrimination

Treating someone less favourably as a result of a 'protected characteristic'.

Indirect Discrimination

Circumstances or requirements that place a person/group of people at a disadvantage.

Victimisation

Treating someone less favourably because they have:

» made or intend to make a complaint or allegation, or

» made or intend to give evidence in relation to a complaint of discrimination.

Harassment

Engaging in unwanted contact towards others that violates dignity or creates an intimidating, hostile or degrading or offensive environment.

Failure to make reasonable adjustment(s)

The Act recognises that the environment can create significant barriers for people; it imposes a specific duty to make reasonable adjustments. The failure to make such reasonable adjustments is considered to be unlawful treatment.

The Human Rights Act (1998)

Human rights are the legal rights which belong to us all, regardless of individual or group differences.

These rights:

» regulate the relationship between the individual and the state by setting the basic standards expected by public authorities;

» were first legally defined by the 1948 Universal Declaration of Human Rights, following the atrocities of the holocaust evidenced at the end of World War 2;

» were adapted to become the European Convention of Human Rights (ECHR), to which the United Kingdom (UK) became a signatory in 1951;

» became enshrined in UK Law in 1998 in the form of the Human Rights Act.

FREDA

The *FREDA* acronym assists in highlighting the founding principles of this Act:

Fairness

Respect

Equality

Dignity

Autonomy

 SnapShot on ... **Mental Capacity Act (2005)**

As evidenced within Serious Case Reviews and Safeguarding Adult Reviews (Table 1.1), there can be situations where a person has the mental capacity to make a required decision at certain times, but lacks this at others; this is described as *fluctuating capacity*.

The Mental Capacity Act (2005) requires that people are supported to make their own decisions whenever this is possible, based upon a clear assessment of their mental capacity to make a decision at the time a decision is required. In cases where a person is assessed to lack the mental capacity to make a specific decision at a specific time, decisions can be made in that person's 'best interests' at that time. At each and every stage of an assessment of an individual's mental capacity, and best-interests decision-making process (as applicable), accurate records, involving all relevant individuals and/or agencies, must be completed and securely stored.

Where a person is confirmed to lack mental capacity in relation to a time-specific issue/decision (this may include fluctuating capacity as discussed above), the requirements of the Mental Capacity Act (2005) apply in terms of Safeguarding Adults, as in all other circumstances. The Mental Capacity Act (2005) is based upon the following five statutory principles (Section 1):

The Mental Capacity Act (2005) five statutory principles:

1. A person must be assumed to have capacity unless it is established that they lack capacity.

2. A person is not to be treated as unable to make a decision unless all practicable steps to help them to do so have been taken without success.

3. A person is not to be treated as unable to make a decision merely because they make an unwise decision.

4. An act done or decision made, under this Act for or on behalf of a person who lacks capacity must be done, or made, in their best interests.

5. Before the act is done, or the decision is made, regard must be had to whether the purpose for which it is needed can be as effectively achieved in a way that is less restrictive of the person's rights and freedom of action.

(Mental Capacity Act 2005)

A person with mental capacity has the right to make decisions which others may consider to be unwise and to do so freely without influence or coercion. In relation to Safeguarding Adults, individuals may well make decision(s) which others consider to be unwise, particularly in relation to factors of self-neglect. A person is entitled to have steps taken to support them through the decision-making process; this can include for example support with communication, and advocacy.

Fluctuating Mental Capacity

Examples of fluctuating capacity can include

someone who has manic depression may have a temporary manic phase which causes them to lack capacity to make financial decisions, leading them to get into debt even though at other times they are perfectly able to manage their money. A person with a psychotic illness may have delusions that affect their capacity to make decisions at certain times but disappear at others. Temporary factors may also affect someone's ability to make decisions. Examples include acute illness, severe pain, the effect of medication, or distress after a death or shock.

... guidance on how to support someone with fluctuating or temporary capacity to make a decision can be found in chapter 3, particularly paragraphs 3.12–3.16. More information about factors that may indicate that a person may regain or develop capacity in the future can be found at paragraph 5.28.

(Mental Capacity Act 2005 – Code of Practice)

Key factors to consider, particularly in practice with people at risk of self-neglect, include the following:

» Does the person's capacity vary at different times of day? – eg morning or evening?; the impacts of some prescribed medicines, drugs or alcohol.

» Address one decision at a time, and consider not only the capacity of the individual to make an informed choice but also their capacity to execute and follow through the actions associated with the decision made.

» Do not impose unnecessary time restraints; a decision may need to be addressed over an extended period of time/occasions, in order that trust is established.

» Avoid discrimination – do not make assumptions about someone's best interests simply on the basis of the person's age, appearance, condition or behaviour.

» Does the person have *all* information relevant to the decision?

» Do they need support to understand the information and weigh in the balance the implications of this information and the decision to be made; some people may prefer or need someone else with them;

» Consider the location at which the decision is to be made.

Cognitive fluctuations, demotivation or impotence

The area of fluctuating capacity and motivation can be described as a tension between the impotence or refusal of some individuals to manage their own personal health, well-being and safety, in simple terms, 'cognitive stuckness' (see Figure 2.4: Cognitive fluctuations, demotivation or impotence), a concept identified by Dr Andrew Heighton (consultant psychiatrist). This state of cognitive fluctuation in self-neglect can expand or contract based upon a spectrum of strengths, resilience and pressures (push and pull factors), such as:

» pressure from external bodies or agencies (for example, Environmental Health, a landlord, the Police, or the perceptions of local neighbours, family or community who apply pressure to local services to intervene);

» peer, parental or familial support provision or withdrawal;

» changes or fluctuations in mental or physical health;

» alcohol or drug abuse;

» perceptions of threat, and the potential triggering of survival behaviours.

Figure 2.4 Cognitive fluctuations, demotivation or impotence

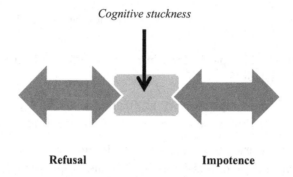

In the context of the tension described above (Figure 2.4) there is also a need to consider any physical health diagnosis which may in the future have an impact upon the person's ability to care for themselves and/or their home environment. The cumulative total of 'refusal' (both historic and current) and the potential future 'impotence' of the individual needs to be considered from a preventative perspective in order to mitigate the risk of an escalation of concerns related to self-neglect.

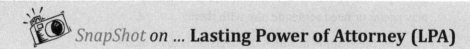

SnapShot on ... Lasting Power of Attorney (LPA)

Lasting Power of Attorney (LPA) is a legal document that enables an individual (the 'donor') to appoint one or more people ('attorneys') to help them to make decisions or to make decisions on their behalf.

There are two types of LPA:

Health and Welfare

This LPA can be used by the donor to give an attorney the power to make decisions about things like:

» Daily routine, for example washing, dressing, eating

» Medical care

» Moving into a care home

» Life-sustaining treatment

It can only be used when the donor is unable to make their own decisions.

Property and Financial Affairs

This LPA can be used to give an attorney the power to make decisions about money and property for the donor, for example:

» Managing a bank or building society account

» Paying bills

» Collecting benefits or a pension

» Selling the donor's home

It can be used as soon as it is registered, with the donor's permission, with the Office of the Public Guardian. One or both of these LPAs can be created by an individual aged 18 years or older – the donor does not need to live in the United Kingdom or be a British Citizen. Different legalities apply in Scotland and Northern Ireland. In order for LPA(s) to be legally recognised they must be registered with the Office of the Public Guardian – details can be found at www.gov.uk/power-of-attorney and Office of the Public Guardian, PO Box 16185, Birmingham, B2 2WH.

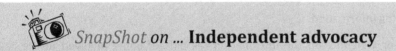

SnapShot on ... **Independent advocacy**

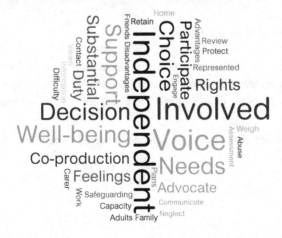

The Oxford Dictionary describes an advocate as *'a person who puts a case on someone else's behalf'.*

Under the Care Act (2014) a person who has 'substantial difficulty' in being included in their care and support processes is entitled to independent advocacy support in order that they are enabled to fully participate. This entitlement equally applies to a need for support with their involvement in any Safeguarding Adults enquiries and/ or investigations.

'advocacy' – supporting a person to understand information, express their needs and wishes, secure their rights, represent their interests and obtain the care and support they need.

(Paragraph 3.9 Care Act Guidance, updated 24 February 2017)

The *two* conditions which must be met for the provision of an independent advocate under the Care Act (2014) are defined as:

1. that if an independent advocate were not provided then the person would have substantial difficulty in being fully involved in these processes;

2. there is no appropriate individual available to support and represent the person's wishes who is not paid or professionally engaged in providing care or treatment to the person or their carer.

What is *substantial difficulty* under the Care Act (2014)?

The concept of 'substantial difficulty' must be judged for each person individually – giving full consideration to each of the *four* areas noted below:

1. understanding relevant information;

2. retaining information;

3. using or weighing up the information (as part of being involved in the key process);

4. communicating their views, wishes and feelings.

Local authorities must consider whether the adult would experience substantial difficulty in any of these 4 areas: understanding the information provided; retaining the information; using or weighing up the information as part of the process of being involved; and communicating the person's views, wishes or feelings.

(paragraph 6.33 Care Act Guidance, updated 24 February 2017)

Links with the Mental Capacity Act (2005):

Where an Independent Mental Capacity Advocate (IMCA) is already involved with an individual then, unless it is inappropriate, the same person/advocate can be used in relation to Care Act procedures.

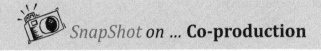

SnapShot on ... **Co-production**

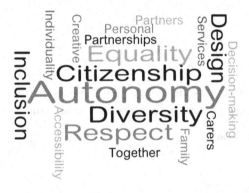

Co-production is a process whereby those who use services and the professionals involved work together as partners:

Some definitions of co-production include:

» A way of working whereby citizens and decision-makers – or people who use services, family carers and service providers – work together to create a decision outcome or service which works for all parties involved. Co-production is value-driven and built on the principle that those who use services are best placed to help design it.

» Co-production is not just a word, it's not just a concept; it is a meeting of minds coming together to find a shared solution to an issue. In practice it involves people who use services being consulted, included and working together from the start to the end of any project that affects them.

» Service users and professionals working together as partners.

(SCIE, 2013)

An example of co-production in action could be a group of service users and professionals creating and distributing materials to raise awareness of adult abuse; how to recognise and report it.

Co-production is different from user involvement; it *'is about developing more equal partnerships between people who use services, carers and professionals'* (SCIE, 2013).

Principles of co-production which are essential values translated into action (Figure 2.5 Principles of co-production):

» Equality

» Diversity

» Accessibility

» Reciprocity

The key concept of *reciprocity* is about ensuring that people receive something back after contributing, and to build upon on a person's desire to feel valued and needed.

Figure 2.5 Principles of co-production

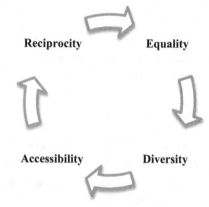

SnapShot on ... **Advance Support Planning**

'Advance Support Planning' has been used extensively within the UK, particularly in the field of palliative care. This approach can prove effective in support of people who have fluctuating and changeable conditions which impact upon their mental capacity to make decisions for themselves (in line with the legal requirements of the Mental Capacity Act (2005); the Mental Health Act (1983); the Human Rights Act (1998)).

In relation to self-neglect, examples of circumstances which impact upon decision-making abilities and mental capacity can include deterioration in a diagnosed mental health condition or the influence of alcohol and/or drug abuse. In order to empower an individual in this circumstance, should they so choose, support in the completion of an *Advance Support Plan* (Table 2.2) at a time when they have the mental capacity to do so, may assist in decision-making when they lack the capacity to do this themselves.

Example components of an 'Advance Support Plan' in self-neglect can include:

» Signs that I may lack capacity;

» What I confirm will help me and has helped me in the past and what hasn't helped me;

» My caring responsibilities at home (this may include children, pets, relatives);

» The arrangements I have in place to assist with my finances;

» The arrangements I have in place to assist with my health and welfare;

» My medication;

» Who I would like to visit me and who I do not want to visit me;

» Further information I feel is important to me when I lack capacity.

Accurate collation of this type of information may be vital in appropriately supporting those people who are receptive to support when they have mental capacity, but become resistant and refuse when they lack capacity. As described previously, tension can lie between the refusal or impotence to act to protect and promote personal well-being and safety.

Illustrative *Example*

A 50-year-old woman, with an enduring mental health condition, experiences fluctuating mental capacity and severely neglects her personal hygiene needs and environment when unwell. This refusal and actual inability to wash and cleanse herself previously resulted in her becoming extremely dirty and unkempt to an extent which posed significant personal and environmental health risks.

Following an extended period of social care involvement she completed her own Advance Support Plan when she was well; this described how she could be supported when she was unwell.

This Advance Support Plan gave her the reassurance that those involved with her would understand more fully who she is and how to work more effectively with her when she becomes unwell and experiences an acute deterioration in her mental health and mental capacity.

Table 2.2 An example format for an *Advance Support Plan*

My Advance Support Plan – CHOICE & CONTROL			
My full name is		**My date of birth is**	
I like to be called			
My address is			
☎ **Telephone**			
✉ **Email**			
This is my 'Advance Support Plan'. I would like this to be used, should I become unwell, to provide information about (TICK as applicable and add further details as applicable in the spaces below): ☐ Signs that I may be becoming unwell ☐ What has helped me in the past ☐ What hasn't helped me ☐ My caring responsibilities at home (this may include children, pets, relatives) ☐ The arrangements I have in place to assist with my finances ☐ The arrangements I have in place to assist with my health and welfare ☐ My medication ☐ Who I would like to visit me ☐ Who I do not want to visit me ☐ .... ☐			
My signature		**Date signed**	
Witnessed by			
Name		**Date signed**	
Signature			
Name		**Date signed**	
Signature			
The names and contact details of Health and Social Care Practitioners who are involved with me are:			
Care coordinator			
Social worker			
GP			
Psychiatrist/ consultant			
Registered nurse			
In the event that this 'Advance Support Plan' is to be used I would like the following person(s) to be contacted:			

My Advance Support Plan – CHOICE & CONTROL		
Name		Relationship to me:
Address		
☎ Telephone		
✉ Email		

These are signs that I have shown in the past when I am becoming unwell

Add your own descriptions here.

These are things that have helped me in the past:

Add your own descriptions here (for example, include treatments, medicines, how people communicate with you, etc).

These are things that have NOT helped me in the past:

Add your own descriptions here (for example, include treatments, medicines, how people communicate with you, etc).

These are my current diagnosed illnesses, and treatment plans:

Add your own descriptions here.

These are the things I need help and support with:

Add your own descriptions here (for example, help with reading and/or writing; physical disabilities; walking; using the toilet; having a shower; making a drink; eating a meal, etc).

When I am well these are my caring responsibilities:

Add your own descriptions here (for example, include if you have children, dependent relatives/friends, pets, etc).

When I am unwell I have made the following arrangements to meet my caring responsibilities:

Add your own descriptions here.

These are the arrangements I have in place to assist me with my finances:

Add your own descriptions here giving the *full* name and contact details (for example, include if you have an Appointee to assist with Welfare Benefits or a Lasting Power of Attorney).

These are the arrangements I have in place to assist me with my health and welfare:

Add your own descriptions here giving the *full* name and contact details (for example, include if you have a Lasting Power of Attorney).

At the time of writing this Advance Support Plan these are the medicines I am taking – PLEASE CHECK THESE DETAILS AT THE TIME THIS ADVANCE SUPPORT PLAN IS TO BE USED:

My Advance Support Plan – CHOICE & CONTROL		
Add your own details here.		
I would be happy if these people visited me when I am unwell:		
Name		**Relationship to me:**
Address		
☎ **Telephone**		
⊠ **Email**		
Name		**Relationship to me:**
Address		
☎ **Telephone**		
⊠ **Email**		
I would NOT like these people to visit me when I am unwell:		
Name		**Relationship to me:**
Address		
☎ **Telephone**		
⊠ **Email**		
Name		**Relationship to me:**
Address		
☎ **Telephone**		
⊠ **Email**		
Further information I feel is important to me when I am unwell:		
Add your own description here.		
I will review this 'Advance Support Plan':		
Add your chosen timescale here; it can be as often as you choose.		
Date planned	**Date review completed**	**Your signature**
I have given a copy of my Advance Support Plan to:		
Name		**Relationship to me:**

This chapter has introduced a structured framework for interventions with people who self-neglect, underpinned by a person-centred approach to risks and strengths assessment. Key issues in this area relate to the need for practitioners to be enabled and supported to consistently recognise and respond proactively to cases where fluctuating capacity and the risk of disengagement are contributory factors in self-neglect, and increase the risk of harm occurring to the person.

Taking it Further

Publications

Briggs, M (September 2013) A six-point guide to how social workers can improve the lives of abused adults. [online] Available at: www.communitycare.co.uk/2013/09/03/a-six-point-guide-to-how-social-workers-can-improve-the-lives-of-abused-adults/

Caldicott, F (1997) *The Caldicott Report on the Review of Patient-identifiable Information*. Department of Health.

Donovan, K and Regehr, C (2010) Elder Abuse: Clinical, Ethical, and Legal Considerations in Social Work Practice. *Journal of Clinical Social Work*, 38: 174–82.

Gálvez-Andres, A, Blasco-Fontecilla, H, González-Parra, S, de Dios Molina, J, Padín, J M and Rodriguez, R H (2007) Secondary Bipolar Disorder and Diogenes Syndrome in Frontotemporal Dementia: Behavioral Improvement with Quetiapine and Sodium Valproate. *Journal of Clinical* Psychopharmacology, 27(6): 722–3.

Macleod, A D (1988). Self-neglect of Spinal Injured Patients. *Paraplegia*, 26(5): 340–9.

McDermott, S, Linahan, K and Squires, B J (2009) Older People Living in Squalor: Ethical and Practical Dilemmas *Australian Social Work*, 62(2): 245–57.

Naik, A D, Lai, J M, Kunik, M E, Dyer, C B (2008) Assessing Capacity in Suspected Cases of Self-neglect. *Geriatrics*, 63(2): 24–31.

O'Connor, D, Hall, M I and Donnelly, M (2009) Assessing Capacity Within a Context of Abuse or Neglect. *Journal of Elder Abuse or* Neglect, 21: 156–69.

Websites

Community Care (2016) A Six-point Guide to How Social Workers Can Improve the Lives of Abused Adults. [online] Available at: www.communitycare.co.uk/2013/09/03/a-six-point-guide-to-how-social-workers-can-improve-the-lives-of-abused-adults/ (accessed 16 May 2017).

UK Government (n.d.) Lasting Power of Attorney, Being in Care and Your Financial Affairs. [online] Available at: www.gov.uk/browse/births-deaths-marriages/lasting-power-attorney (accessed 16 May 2017).

Other sources

Office of the Public Guardian, PO Box 16185, Birmingham, B2 2WH.

References

Department for Children, Schools and Families, and Communities and Local Government (2008) *Information Sharing: Guidance for Practitioners and Managers.*

Department of Health (2017) *The Care and Support Statutory Guidance.*

SCIE (2013) *Co-Production in Social Care: What It Is and How to Do It.* (Guide 51).

The Stationery Office on behalf of the Department for Constitutional Affairs (2007) *The Mental Capacity Act Code of Practice.*

West of Berkshire Safeguarding Adults Board (2016) Safeguarding Adult Review Mr I. [online] Available at: www.hampshiresab.org.uk/wp-content/uploads/SAR-Mr-I-Final-Report-2016v4.pdf (accessed 16 May 2017).

Introduction

In this chapter we detail our model for risks and strengths assessment in self-neglect. This is supported by full guidance notes, illustrative examples and sample document formats, including *SnapShots* that summarise some key areas for consideration which build on those given in previous chapters:

» driving and restraining forces to consider when utilising a conceptual risk assessment model – a human perspective;

» criminal offences and safeguarding adults;

» domestic abuse;

» The Modern Slavery Act (2015);

» exploitation and illegal drug use;

» grooming;

» mate crime.

Figure 3.1 The Risks and Strengths Balance

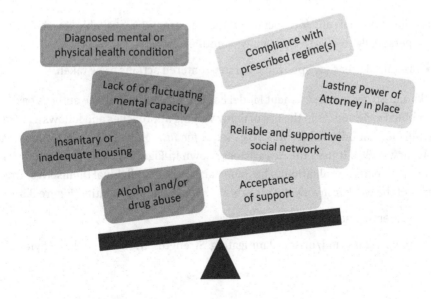

'Risk assessment' is a traditionally recognised term to describe the:

» identification of known or potentially hazardous, risky issues, circumstances or relationships;

» impact or consequence of the hazard/risk;

» likelihood that the identified hazard/risk will occur.

The personalisation agenda requires that the adult at risk is at the centre of *all* interventions, and that they are supported to live their chosen lifestyle.

Living life is not risk free!

Taking a Risks and Strengths Balance (Figure 3.1) approach to assessment and support planning in Safeguarding enables:

» an evaluation of potential and/or actual risk factors associated with an individual;

» the identification of their personal and/or social strengths which mitigate those risks;

» the person to be at the centre and in control wherever and whenever possible (based upon individual needs, circumstances and legal requirements).

The suggested Risks and Strengths Assessment Model in cases of self-neglect uses the Key Factors shown in Figure 3.2 below as a framework for individual, person-centred evaluation to be undertaken by the individual themselves wherever possible, and the worker involved. This process should initially identify:

» presenting actual or potential risks;

» the personal and/or social mitigating strengths available to the individual personally to effectively manage identified risks;

» required areas for applicable person-centered actions to be taken.

This Risks and Strengths Assessment Model has been developed by the authors based upon their combined experiences in the use of many varying approaches and follows a red, amber, green (RAG) format adapted from *A Risk Matrix for Risk Managers* (NHS National Patient Safety Agency, 2008). It uses the Key Factors shown in Figure 3.2 as a framework for individual, person-centred evaluation to be undertaken by the individual themselves, wherever possible, and the worker involved. This process should initially identify (Figure 3.3):

» presenting actual or potential risks;

» the personal and/or social mitigating 'Strengths' available to the individual.

Figure 3.2 Key factors in self-neglect

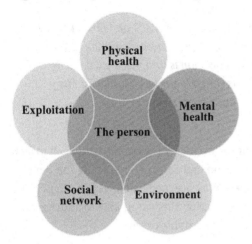

Case Study: Community Assets and Strengths

Mary is 80 years old and lives alone in a privately owned property; she has maintained an extremely private lifestyle, she has no close family and hasn't let anyone into her home for several years. Mary visits her local church each week (across the road) and presents positively when out in the community, but lives at home in insanitary conditions. The condition of Mary's home includes infestation by rodents and insects (moths), as well as the lack of a flushing toilet (due to a longstanding blockage), and 'clutter' which prevents her from accessing her kitchen and bathroom/toilet. Mary has been disposing urine and faeces in the drain in her backyard for at least two years. The infestation and stench is impacting upon her neighbours who have reported their concerns to the local authority.

A home visit is made to Mary, where the actual and potential risks to her and her neighbours' health, well-being and safety are identified with her. Mary finds this home visit difficult, but she cooperates, and with sensitive discussion accepts the need to address the risks/hazards. Mary decides to take action with support from her local church.

With support Mary has shown the personal and social 'strength' to address concerns, and actually requires minimal intervention from statutory agencies. A Support Plan is developed and agreed with Mary and her local church to 'de-clutter' and clean her home, and to immediately arrange for the repair of the blocked toilet and de-infestation. While the property is de-infested and the toilet is repaired Mary stays with a church member.

Summary:

The presenting risks/hazards score HIGH both in terms of IMPACT and LIKELIHOOD; however, with the inclusion of Mary's 'strength', which evidences mitigating factors, this is significantly reduced. A review of the Support Plan is completed, all agreed actions have been completed and the concern is closed to the local authority. Mary was relieved, and is now continuing to ask for and accept support.

The above Case Study shows that what may appear to be a highly serious situation can in fact be sensitively managed to maximise self-determination and control by keeping the person at the centre of all interventions. In this case the person concerned had always been private and independent; she had simply found herself in a situation she was unable to address and her circumstances had deteriorated to a potentially catastrophic extent.

Figure 3.3 Person-centred planning

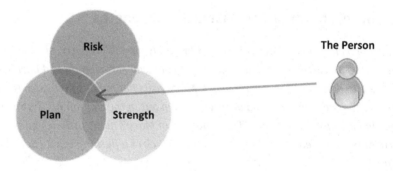

How to use this Model:

The allocated case assessor should consider each of the *Key Factors* included within Table 3.1 and individually measure their potential *IMPACT* upon the adult at risk. It should be noted that Table 3.1 is not an exhaustive or exclusive list, and professional judgement should be used to accurately reflect the individual adult at risk and their circumstances:

1. *ACTUAL RISK*: A brief summary should be added to the *ACTUAL RISK* column of the Risks and Strengths Assessment Model to confirm identified concerns.

2. *IMPACT*: Using Table 3.2, the applicable Risk Level Score should be added to the *IMPACT* (I) column of the Risks and Strengths Assessment Model.

3. *LIKELIHOOD*: Using Table 3.3, the applicable Risk Level Score should then be added to the *LIKELIHOOD* (L) column.

The Risks and Strengths Assessment Model will then calculate the *RISK GRADING* of each *Key Factor* (Table 3.4 IMPACT × LIKELIHOOD = Risk Grading).

Based upon the Risk Factors identified and their overarching *GRADING* the allocated case assessor should, for each *Key Factor*, confirm within the Risks and Strengths Assessment Model (Table 3.5):

» actions to be taken;

» the timescale within which these will be completed;

» the Agency or individual responsible.

Following implementation of a *Self-neglect* Safeguarding Support Plan, as applicable to each individual case, the Risks and Strengths Assessment Model should be used at the point of each *REVIEW* in order to evidence progress in the management and mitigation of risk, and as a basis for future Support Plans.

Table 3.1 The Risks and Strengths Balance

Key Factor	Description/Prompts
Mental Health	Diagnosed Mental Health condition, learning difficulties and/or impaired cognition, including Diogenes syndrome.
	Recent deterioration in mental health state (may include the lack of motivation to meet essential personal care needs, recent loss/bereavement, and/or traumatic event).
	Involvement with specialist healthcare professionals.
	Non-concordance with treatment plan and/or prescribed medication regime.
	Lack of or fluctuating mental capacity to make informed decisions in this regard, following assessment in line with the requirements of the Mental Capacity Act (2005).
	Known pattern of problematic alcohol use/dependency.
	Known pattern of illegal substance misuse.
	Involvement with the Police and/or Probation Service (may include MAPPA).
Physical Health	Recognised 'Long-term/Enduring Condition' for which treatment/medicine is prescribed.
	Long-term/Enduring Condition which has the potential to reduce life expectancy if not managed.
	Deterioration in physical health state and/or exacerbation of existing condition.
	Involvement with specialist healthcare professionals.
	Non-concordance with treatment plan and/or prescribed medication regime.

Key Factor	Description/Prompts
Housing	Non-secure tenure – may be assured shorthold *or* informal arrangement (this can include for example bed and breakfast accommodation and/or 'sofa-surfing').
	Not suitable to meet needs – mobility or environmental factors.
	Inadequate essential amenities (utilities).
	Refusal to engage with support agencies.
	Insanitary conditions and/or hoarding (objects and/or animals), which will lead to the involvement of Environmental Health Services and may also include Fire Services.
Social Network/ Lifestyle Choices	Relationships – which may be problematic, hazardous and/or abusive (including alcohol/substance dependencies).
	Children and/or other adults at risk living at the property.
	Limited/no reliable social network of family/friends *and/or* risks posed by a carer.
	Known pattern of involvement with the criminal justice system.
	Known pattern of involvement with statutory agencies (including crisis intervention).
	Homelessness.
	Debt with inadequate resources to meet demands.
	Involvement with the Police and/or Probation Service (may include MAPPA).
	Young adults at risk in Transition from Children to Adult Social Care Services.
Exploitation/ Abuse	Involvement with statutory agencies regarding allegations of abuse (in line with Safeguarding Adults definition).
	Known involvement with criminal justice offenders and/or perpetrators of abuse.
	Low self-esteem/worth.
	'Attention-seeking' behaviours which are potentially hazardous (eg attachment disorders).
	Changes in usual routines, refusal to discuss the basis or nature of these changes.
	Deterioration in 'usual' personal presentation; this may include physical signs of assault and/or withdrawal from engagement/involvement.
	Involvement with the Police and/or Probation Service (may include MAPPA).
	Young adults at risk in Transition from Children to Adult Social Care Services.
Adverse Publicity/ Damage to the Reputation of the Agency and Public Confidence	Rumours; potential for public concern.
	Local, short-term media coverage – minimal public concern.
	Local media-coverage – long-term reduction in public confidence.
	National media coverage – long-term reduction in public confidence.
	National media coverage which includes the attention of the local parliamentary representative and a total loss of public confidence.
	Complaint which may include referral and/or investigation by the Ombudsman.
	Criteria for a Safeguarding Adults Review may be met.
	Potential for Litigation; criminal prosecution.
	Breach(es) in statutory duty.
	MAPPA arrangements.

Table 3.2 Impact score – level of severity

KEY Factor	Risk Level				
	1	**2**	**3**	**4**	**5**
	Negligible	**Low**	**Moderate**	**High**	**Critical/Immediate**
1. Mental Health	No associated known risk factors	Identified/associated risk is managed effectively by the individual themselves with no on-going support services required.	Identified/associated risk is managed effectively but will deteriorate without on-going and consistent support from social and/or healthcare professionals – this may result in harm occurring.	Identified/associated risk is not effectively managed; there are no support mechanisms in place or operational, no cooperation with support, treatment and/or medication plans – harm may occur to the individual if support is not arranged and accepted. Admission to hospital or alternative accommodation (eg care home/respite care) may be required.	Immediate and critical risk to the safety of the adult at risk and/ or others (eg children and/or other adults at risk who reside at the property); may include an assessment under the requirements of the Mental Health Act 1983 and/or the involvement of the Police.
2. Physical Health					
3. Housing	No associated known risk factors	The environment is 'cluttered' and untidy but does not pose a risk of harm or to safety. There is no threat of homelessness or harm. Signposting/ referral to support/ advice services (including as applicable financial advice, cleaning services, etc) is required. The adult at risk is cooperative.	The environment shows evidence of problematic hoarding to an extent which could result in risk to health, safety and/ or homelessness if not effectively managed. The environment will deteriorate without on-going and consistent support from social care, housing support or Environmental Health professionals as applicable. The adult at risk is cooperative.	No effective support mechanisms are in place or operational. The home environment shows evidence of the problematic hoarding of both objects and animals. Homelessness is threatened; eviction may be planned. Admission to alternative accommodation (eg care home/respite care) may be required. Input from social/ health care, housing support, Animal Welfare (eg RSPCA) and/or Environmental Health professionals is required as applicable. Fire Service. The adult at risk is non-cooperative.	Immediate and critical risk to the safety of the adult at risk and/ or others (eg children and/or other adults at risk who reside at the property) and may include the involvement of the Police.

	Risk Level				
	1	2	3	4	5
4. Social Network	No associated known risk factors.	The adult at risk has a supportive social network and/or informal carers but requires information, advice and support particularly in relation to applicable welfare benefits and local support services – this will include voluntary sector organisations(s).	The adult at risk has a support network which is at risk of breakdown; factors may include debt, carer stress, problematic alcohol and drug dependencies. The adult at risk has a history of involvement with the Police and/or Probation Service. Carer Assessment and input from specialist support services are required.	The adult at risk is directly and consistently involved with hazardous and problematic relationships. Abuse from/to the adult at risk is reported; there is no reliable or safe support network. Police involvement is frequent, and continues to be required. Specialist support services are required.	Immediate and critical risk to the safety of the adult at risk and/or others (eg children and/or other adults at risk who reside at the property); includes the involvement of the Police.
5. Exploitation/ Abuse	No associated known risk factors.	The adult at risk has low self-esteem, and a sense of self-worth. They are vulnerable to negative influences and attention; however, a positive, effective and vigilant support network is in place. Signposting/referral to local voluntary/third-sector organisations may provide additional social support.	The adult at risk has low self-esteem, and a sense of self-worth. They are vulnerable to negative influences and attention due to their own lack of insight into risk and the potentially abusive and hazardous motivations of others. The individual is cooperative with all agencies, and shows no known signs or symptoms of abuse or radicalisation.	The adult at risk has previous involvement with statutory agencies in relation to abuse perpetrated by others. The adult at risk is known to con-tinue to be in close contact with their abusers. The individual is reluctant to or has refused to cooperate with support services. The involvement of the Police and specialist services is required.	Immediate and critical risk to the safety of the adult at risk and/or others (eg children and/or other adults at risk who reside at the property), and includes the involvement of the Police with other applicable specialist support services.

	Risk Level				
	1	2	3	4	5
6. Adverse Publicity/ Damage to the Reputation of the Agency and Public Confidence	Negative rumours. Minimal potential for media interest.	Local media involved – short-term adverse publicity.\n\nRisk Assessment and Management Support Plans are robust.	Local media attention, complaint submitted or likely to be submitted.\n\nOn-going adverse media attention which has/will reduce public confidence.\n\nInadequately documented Risk Assessment and/ or Management Support Plans *and* no clear decision-making process recorded.\n\nProbation Service and/or MAPPA may be involved.	Complainant not satisfied with response. Ombudsman is or is likely to be involved.\n\nKnown reduction in public confidence – no recorded/documented Risk Assessment and/or Management Support Plans *and* no decision-making process.\n\nRisk of criminal prosecution(s).\n\nRisk of breach(es) in statutory duty.	Immediate risk of death or serious harm suffered by an adult at risk, or child.\n\nTotal loss of public confidence.\n\nSAR Criteria met.\n\nBreach(es) in statutory duty.\n\nThreat of criminal prosecution(s)

Table 3.3 Likelihood score – frequency

Factors	Risk Level				
	1	2	3	4	5
Descriptor	Rare	Unlikely	Possible	Likely	Almost certain
Frequency How often might it/does it happen?	This will probably never happen/ recur	Do not expect it to happen/ recur but it is possible it may do so	Might happen or recur occasionally	Will probably happen/recur, but it is not a persisting issue/ circumstance	Will undoubtedly happen/ recur, possibly frequently

Table 3.4 Risk 'grading' – by key factor (IMPACT × LIKELIHOOD = GRADING)

IMPACT	LIKELIHOOD				
	1	2	3	4	5
	Rare	Unlikely	Possible	Likely	Almost certain
5 Critical/ Immediate	5	10	15	20	25
4 High	4	8	12	16	20
3 Moderate	3	6	9	12	15
2 Low	2	4	6	8	10
1 Negligible	1	2	3	4	5

Risk Grading Summary:
1–3: LOW RISK
4–6: MODERATE RISK
8–12: HIGH RISK
15–25: CRITICAL/IMMEDIATE RISK

Table 3.5 Self-neglect – Risks and Strengths Assessment Model

Name of Adult at Risk:	
Unique Identifier:	
Risk Assessment completed by:	
Date Risk Assessment completed:	

KEY FACTOR	DESCRIPTION/PROMPTS	ACTUAL RISKS	Impact	Likelihood	Grading	ACTIONS TO BE TAKEN	TIMESCALE	RESPONSIBLE PERSON/ AGENCY
Mental Health	Diagnosed Mental Health condition, learning difficulties and/or impaired cognition, including Diogenes and/or Noah syndrome. Recent deterioration in mental health state (may include the lack of motivation to meet essential personal care needs, recent loss/bereavement, and/or traumatic event). Involvement with specialist healthcare professional. Non-concordance with treatment plan and/or prescribed medication regime.							
	Lack of or fluctuating mental capacity to make informed decisions in this regard, following assessment in line with the requirements of the Mental Capacity Act (2005). Known pattern of problematic alcohol use/dependency. Known pattern of illegal substance misuse. Involvement with the Police and/or Probation Service (may include MAPPA).							

Name of Adult at Risk:

KEY FACTOR	DESCRIPTION/PROMPTS	ACTUAL RISKS	Impact	Likelihood	Grading	ACTIONS TO BE TAKEN	TIMESCALE	RESPONSIBLE PERSON/AGENCY
Physical Health	Recognised Long-term/Enduring Condition for which treatment/medicine is prescribed.							
	Long-term/Enduring Condition which has the potential to reduce life expectancy if not managed.							
	Deterioration in physical health state and/or exacerbation of existing condition.							
	Involvement with specialist healthcare professional.							
	Non-concordance with treatment plan and/or prescribed medication regime.							
Housing	Non-secure tenure – may be assured shorthold *or* informal arrangement (this can include for example bed and breakfast accommodation and/or 'sofa-surfing').							
	Not suitable to meet needs – mobility or environmental factors.							
	Inadequate essential amenities (utilities).							
	Refusal to engage with support agencies.							
	Insanitary conditions and/or hoarding (objects and/or animals), which will lead to the involvement of Environmental Health Services and may also include Fire Services.							
Social Network	Relationships – which may be problematic, hazardous and/or abusive (including alcohol/substance dependencies).							
	Children and/or other adults at risk living at the property.							
	Limited/no reliable social network of family/friends *and/or* risks posed by a carer.							

Name of Adult at Risk:				
	Known pattern of involvement with the criminal justice system.			
	Known pattern of involvement with statutory agencies (including crisis intervention).			
	Homelessness.			
	Debt with inadequate resources to meet demands.			
	Involvement with the Police and/or Probation Service (may include MAPPA).			
	Young adults at risk in Transition from Children to Adult Social Care Services.			
Exploitation/ Abuse	Involvement with statutory agencies regarding allegations of abuse (in line with Safeguarding Adults definition).			
	Known involvement with criminal justice offenders and/or perpetrators of abuse.			
	Low self-esteem/worth.			
	'Attention-seeking' behaviours which are potentially hazardous (eg attachment disorders).			
	Changes in usual routines, refusal to discuss the basis or nature of these changes.			
	Deterioration in 'usual' personal presentation; this may include physical signs of assault and/or withdrawal from engagement/involvement.			
	Involvement with the Police and/or Probation Service (may include MAPPA).			
	Young adults at risk in Transition from Children to Adult Social Care Services.			

Name of Adult at Risk:								
KEY FACTOR	DESCRIPTION/PROMPTS	ACTUAL RISKS	Impact	Likelihood	Grading	ACTIONS TO BE TAKEN	TIMESCALE	RESPONSIBLE PERSON/AGENCY
Organisational	Rumours; potential for public concern. Local, short-term media coverage – minimal public concern. Local media-coverage – long-term reduction in public confidence. National media coverage – long-term reduction in public confidence. National media coverage which includes the attention of the local parliamentary representative and a total loss of public confidence. Complaint which may include referral and/or investigation by the Ombudsman. Criteria for a Safeguarding Adults Review may be met. Potential for Litigation; criminal prosecution. Breach(es) in statutory duty MAPPA arrangements.							

Practice matters ...

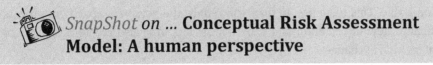

SnapShot on ... **Conceptual Risk Assessment Model: A human perspective**

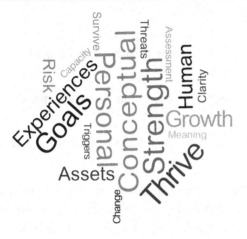

Driving and restraining forces to consider when utilising

a Conceptual Risks and Strengths Assessment Model:

a human perspective

Any intervention to support a person who is self-neglecting or is at risk of self-neglect will inevitably be challenging. The intervention may well be perceived as a 'threat' to the person concerned, as well as an opportunity for potential personal growth and life-enhancing change. As humans we have a tendency to focus more acutely on 'threats' to our personal survival; this predisposition may pose significant challenges for any professional involved in supporting a person who is self-neglecting, or is at risk of self-neglect.

Evolutionary perspective

Humans have evolved to be very sensitive to perceived threats in their own environment – 'survival instinct':

» Flight;

» Fight;

» Freeze.

In general, a situation which is perceived to be 'too different' can, for some, equate to a 'threat to their survival'. It is therefore essential to ensure that any intervention considers and incorporates this factor. Being faced with 'too much difference' can trigger a person's survival instinct to keep themselves and their environment safe and stable. This response, in turn, can reduce the person's capacity to process and manage new information and experiences; this may also create resistance to any suggestion of change.

Roles and goals

Each and every intervention should be based upon clear and specific *goals*, in order to establish a context. These can be expressed as:

» *Explicit goals:* eg to create a safe sleeping environment within a home which is extremely cluttered.

» *Implicit goals:* eg to survive, to keep the situation stable versus to grow and develop.

If the *explicit* goal to be achieved is not clearly specified and understood, there is an increased risk of triggering the *implicit* goal to survive, and thus progress will be impeded and create challenges for both the person at the centre of the intervention and the person supporting them.

As humans we need meaning; the following simple questions are useful in establishing reasons for change:

» *What* is the reason for doing things this way?

» *Why* do things need to change?

If roles are not clear, *how* does the person at the centre of the intervention know what they need to do? They may believe that someone else is responsible for the action; this in itself may meet their personal *implicit goal* to convince themselves that the required action is someone else's job/responsibility.

Survive or thrive?

The ability to keep a person receptive to new experiences is a vital component of the successful navigation of positive change and to achieve 'the best' out of a situation a person may not necessarily want to fully embrace.

The person at the centre of the intervention may react against the authority held by the person responsible for the instigation of necessary change. Resistance to change can be *triggered* by many and varying factors; for example:

> » An instruction or request;
> » Tone of voice, word choice, 'a saying';
> » Facial expression, a gesture.

The person may react in compliance or act defiantly; both of these are survival responses and are likely to come from a place where the person is less able to learn and develop from the process. These are both normal human reactions – 'Don't take it personally'.

Impact?

The complexity of managing human interactions, especially in situations where a person is severely self-neglecting, can *open up* gaps in information-sharing; this in itself can potentially lead to increased risk:

> » Delays in decision-making;
> » Factors/information missed;
> » People being invalidated;
> » Complaints and Safeguarding Concerns being raised;
> » It is a virtual 'minefield';
> » Technical solutions rarely solve non-technical problems;
> » It is difficult to devise an Action Plan that encompasses values and feelings.

Summary:

Supporting a person who self-neglects, or is at risk of self-neglect, is a highly complex Human Event, even in what may appear to be the most straightforward of circumstances. People in these situations are more likely to have experienced trauma, may have reduced capacity to tolerate change, and have developed unhelpful survival behaviours as a result of their personal experiences.

Acknowledgement:

Adapted from a presentation given by Dr Andrew Heighton (MBChB, MRCPsych) September 2017; given with acknowledgement to the many works of the late psychologist Yvonne M Agazarian (Agazarian, Y and Porter Gantt, S (2002) *Autobiography of a Theory of Living Human Systems and Its Systems-centered Practice*. London: Jessica Kingsley Publishers.

SnapShot *on* ... **Criminal offences and safeguarding adults**

In cases where a criminal offence may have taken place, although the local authority takes a lead role it is important to involve the Police as a matter of urgency. This is vital for many reasons, not least that forensic evidence may need to be gathered.

Whether or not a criminal act is committed does not depend on the consent of the victim. Criminal investigation by the police takes priority over all other enquiries but not over the adult's well-being. Close cooperation and coordination among the relevant agencies is critical to ensure safety and well-being is promoted during any criminal investigation process.

(*Care and Support Statutory Guidance*, 2017)

The Care Act Statutory Guidance (Chapter 14) contains details of legal requirements in relation to Safeguarding Adults and case examples for reference; the Youth Justice and Criminal Evidence Act (1999) Part 11, Chapter 1 defines 'special measures directions in case of vulnerable and intimidated witnesses'.

Initial considerations if a crime is suspected

Where it is clear a crime has been committed the *police must be contacted immediately.*

To enable the Police to investigate effectively it is vital that essential evidence is not destroyed or contaminated:

» Immediately contact the Police.

» Do not clean up the scene, touch or remove anything.

» Do not get the victim to bathe or wash. Remember the victim and the alleged perpetrator are part of the scene of crime too and they should not destroy or contaminate evidence.

» Do not touch any weapons – leave them where they are.

» Do not let anyone into the area – if it is a room (bedroom, toilet, etc) shut the door and lock it if possible.

» Do not arrange for a medical examination; the Police will arrange this. The Police may ask for photographs to be taken if there is a camera available.

» Do not have physical contact with the victim or alleged perpetrator as cross-contamination can destroy evidence.

Remember

» The Police are the experts – they will tell you what to do.

» In cases of criminal investigation follow the directions of the Police and do not contaminate or prejudice their investigation.

The process

The Police will investigate an alleged crime and determine whether or not it should be referred to the Crown Prosecution Service (CPS).

In order for a case to go to court, the Crown Prosecution Service consider the evidence and public interest factors, as well as all other applicable legal requirements, for example (taken from *The Code for Crown Prosecutors, 2013. Issued by the Director of Public Prosecutions (DPP) under section 10 of the Prosecution of Offences Act 1985*):

» Can the evidence be used in court?

» Is the evidence reliable and credible?

» How serious is the offence?

» What is the level of culpability of the suspect?

» What are the circumstances of and the harm caused to the victim?

» Was the suspect under the age of 18 at the time of the offence?

» What is the impact upon the community?

» Is prosecution a proportionate response?

» Do sources of information require protecting?

Examples of applicable legislation

» Offences against the Person Act (1861)

» Theft Act (1968)

» Race Relations Act (1976)

» Mental Health Act (1983)

» Police and Criminal Evidence Act (1984)

» Criminal Justice Act (1988)

» Protection from Harassment Act (1997)

» The Crime and Disorder Act (1998)

» Sexual Offences Act (2003)

- » Domestic Violence and Criminal Evidence Act (2004)

- » Mental Capacity Act (2005)

- » The Care Act (2014)

- » The Modern Slavery Act (2015)

- » The Psychoactive Substances Act (2016)

NB: The information and examples given above are not exhaustive and are not designed in any way to constitute legal advice, which should be sought as required.

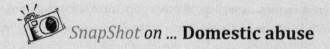 *SnapShot on …* **Domestic abuse**

The Crown Prosection Service Guidelines include the following:

The Government revised its definition of domestic violence and abuse in March 2013 as:

Any incident or pattern of incidents of controlling coercive or threatening behaviour, violence or abuse between those aged 16 or over who are or have been intimate partners or family members, regardless of gender or sexuality.

This can encompass, but is not limited to, the following types of abuse:

- » *psychological;*

- » *physical;*

- » *sexual;*

- » *financial;*

- » *emotional.*

Controlling behaviour *is a range of acts designed to make a person subordinate and/or dependant by isolating them from sources of support, exploiting their resources and capacities for personal gain, depriving them of the means needed for independence, resistance and escape and regulating their everyday behaviour.*

Coercive behaviour *is an act or a pattern of acts of assaults, threats, humiliation and intimidation or other abuse that is used to harm, punish, or frighten their victim.*

(Crown Prosecution Service, 2014)

The definition is supported by an explanatory text:

This definition, which is not a legal definition, includes so called 'honour' based violence, female genital mutilation (FGM) and forced marriage, and is clear that victims are not confined to one gender or ethnic group.

(www.cps.gov.uk)

Domestic abuse is not gender specific and occurs in all cultures. People of all races, ethnicities, religions, ages, sexual orientation and identity can experience domestic abuse; its potential effects are described in Table 3.6 below:

Table 3.6 Effects of Domestic Abuse

Effects of Domestic Abuse can include (not an exhaustive list):		
EMOTIONAL	**PHYSICAL**	**SOCIAL**
Changes in mood	Death	Loss of employment
Chronic anxiety	Injury	Deprivation
Stress	Disability	Alienation
Self-hatred	Fatigue	Family break-up
Lack of interest or enjoyment in life	Self-harm	Disconnection from social norms
Suicidal thinking	Suicide attempts	
Fear and anger	Palpitations	
Loss of libido	Sleep disturbance	

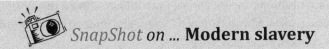

SnapShot on ... **Modern slavery**

The Modern Slavery Act (2015) received Royal Assent on 26th March 2015. This Act of Parliament defines the current definition of 'modern slavery', the legal context and how prevention and protection for victims will be pursued to tackle perpetrators. Since March 2015 the majority of provisions in this Act have come into force in England and Wales. The Act enhances and formalises actions to be taken in order that the criminal justice system effectively prosecutes criminals and protects victims of slavery and/or trafficking.

Slavery, servitude and forced or compulsory labour

An individual's consent to the conduct alleged to amount to slavery, servitude or forced or compulsory labour does not prevent the offence being committed. This provision could be particularly relevant in cases where the victim is vulnerable to abuse, for example a child.

(Home Office Circular, July 2015)

Human trafficking

... where a person arranges or facilitates the travel of another person with a view to that other person being exploited ... it is irrelevant whether or not the victim consents.

(Home Office Circular, July 2015)

This includes the 'intent' to commit a criminal offence.

Exploitation

This includes: slavery, servitude and forced or compulsory labour; sexual exploitation; removal of organs; securing services etc by force, threats or deception; and securing services etc from children and vulnerable persons

(Home Office Circular, July 2015)

Defence for Victims

Section 45 of the Act provides

for a defence for victims of slavery or trafficking who have committed a criminal offence. The defence is intended to provide further encouragement to victims to come forward and give evidence without fear of being prosecuted and *convicted for offences connected to their slavery or trafficking situation.*

(Home Office Circular, July 2015)

All sectors, agencies, organisations and individual practitioners have a responsibility to be aware of the issues associated with Modern Slavery and understand how to recognise and report any concerns that may arise

Freeing the nation from these cruel acts is a responsibility for us all and a priority for the government.

(Modern Slavery: a briefing www.modernslavery.co.uk).

The duty to notify

The *duty to notify* of suspected cases of modern slavery is placed upon all frontline workers involved with vulnerable adults and children; this is done via the Police or the National Referral Mechanism (NRM), dependent upon local procedures – full details will be available from employers and can be found at www.gov.uk, www. modernslavery.co.uk and the helpline: 0800 0121 700.

Identifying victims – useful questions (Salvation Army: 'Spot the Signs')

» Is the victim in possession of a passport, identification or travel documents? Are these documents in possession of someone else?

» Does the victim act as if they were instructed or coached by someone else? Do they allow others to speak for them when spoken to directly?

» Was the victim recruited for one purpose and forced to engage in some other job? Was their transport paid for by facilitators, whom they must pay back through providing services?

» Does the victim receive little or no payment for their work? Is someone else in control of their earnings?

» Was the victim forced to perform sexual acts?

» Does the victim have freedom of movement?

» Has the victim or family been threatened with harm if the victim attempts to escape?

» Is the victim under the impression they are bonded by debt, or in a situation of dependence?

» Has the victim been harmed or deprived of food, water, sleep, medical care or other life necessities?

» Can the victim freely contact friends or family? Do they have limited social interaction or contact with people outside their immediate environment?

 SnapShot on ... **Exploitation and illegal drug use**

The Modern Slavery Act (2015) – as described above – enhances and formalises actions to be taken in order that the criminal justice system effectively prosecutes criminals and protects victims of slavery and/or trafficking.

This includes: slavery, servitude and forced or compulsory labour; sexual exploitation; removal of organs; securing services etc by force, threats or deception; and securing services etc from children and vulnerable persons

(Home Office Circular, July 2015)

Press reports have included the BBC Panorama documentary *Behind Bars: Prison Uncovered* (13 February 2017) and an article in *The Independent*, 'Deadly "legal highs" can now be "ordered like a takeaway" because of government ban, users say' (2 December 2016). Both covered issues surrounding the availability and use of illegal drug substances following the implementation of the Psychoactive Substances Act (2016) which came into force from 26 May 2016 in the UK. This Act of Parliament makes it an offence to produce, supply, offer to supply, possess with intent to supply, possess on custodial premises, import or export psychoactive substances; that is, any substance intended for human consumption that is capable of producing a psychoactive effect.

Of particular interest, and matter of concern, is the relationship between self-neglect, exploitation of 'vulnerable persons' and the supply/use of illegal drugs and substances (also known as New Psychoactive Substances – NPS). There is little, if any, formal research into this relationship; however, based upon our practice experience there exists both a clear cause for concern and need for greater understanding of this issue.

Under the Care Act (2014), local authorities have new functions. This is to make sure that people who live in their areas:

» receive services that prevent their care needs from becoming more serious, or delay the impact of their needs;

» can get the information and advice they need to make good decisions about care and support;

» have a range of provision of high quality, appropriate services to choose from.

In work with adults who are experiencing abuse or neglect *or* are at risk of this occurring, it is important to fully consider the complex issue of self-neglect in terms of the potential impacts of:

» The Modern Slavery Act: is the person being exploited by the securing of services from them?

» The Psychoactive Substances Act: is the person being used as a 'guinea pig' to test out the effects of newly chemically created psychoactive substances?

The hypothesis posed here is that there are causal links between the factors highlighted in Figure 3.4 below, which compound and exacerbate the risk of serious harm occurring.

Figure 3.4 Potential causational links

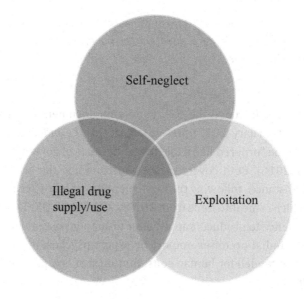

SnapShot on ... **Grooming**

Perpetrators 'groom' a person for the purpose of exploitation in a process designed to break down existing personal defences and relationships to establish control. The purpose of exploitation and control is wide ranging and can include sexual activities, financial gain to criminal activities, including the 'testing of street drugs'.

'Grooming' is a process well recognised in relation to children, but which also impacts upon and victimises adults, particularly those who are vulnerable and/or 'at risk'. Survivors Manchester is a registered charity which works to support adult survivors of abuse, and is part of The Survivors Trust. Survivors Manchester describe adult grooming typically as a process whereby the following practices are used to gain control over another person for the purposes of exploitation.

» *Positive reinforcement*: includes praise, superficial charm, superficial sympathy (crocodile tears), excessive apologising, money, approval, gifts, attention, facial expressions such as a forced laugh or smile, public recognition.

» *Negative reinforcement*: includes nagging, yelling, the silent treatment (sulking), intimidation, threats, swearing, emotional blackmail, the guilt trap, sulking, crying, and playing the victim.

» *Intermittent or partial reinforcement*: to create an effective climate of fear and doubt, for example in terrorist attacks. Partial or intermittent positive reinforcement can encourage the victim to persist; for example in most forms of gambling, the gambler is likely to win now and again but still loses money overall.

» *Punishment.*

» *Traumatic One-Trial Learning*: using verbal abuse, explosive anger, or other intimidating behaviour to establish dominance or superiority; even one incident of such behaviour can condition or train victims to avoid upsetting, confronting or contradicting the manipulator.

» *Normalisation of behaviour.*

(Survivors Manchester, n.d.)

Working with adults at risk and their carers requires the worker to have an awareness of grooming, and to understand how to recognise indicators of this form of abuse. Individuals at risk of grooming may particularly include those people who have learning difficulties, those with mental health problems, and others with low self-esteem and self-worth who may be socially isolated (this is not an exhaustive list as there is no atypical victim type). Workers should also consider if the Serious Crime Act (2015) applies in relation to controlling and coercive behaviours as advised by the

'Controlling or Coercive Behaviour in an Intimate or Family Relationship Statutory Guidance Framwork,' published by the Home Office in December 2015 (Home Office, 2015).

Making Safeguarding Personal requires that the individual themselves is kept at the centre of all Safeguarding enquiries; workers should be sensitive to the possibility of grooming and the exertion of control for exploitative purposes. Examples of this can include the following:

» the forced prostitution of a woman with learning difficulties, which included pornographic filming for sale to others;

» the *testing* of illegal drugs/substances on a man with mental health problems by *street dealers* prior to sale to others – to establish the *safety or impact* of the substances;

» the misuse of, and theft from, a bank account by the family carer of an older person;

» the direction and requirement to commit criminal offences, such as burglary and theft, given to a person with mental health problems by a criminal gang he viewed as his friends;

» the extortion of money and/or property;

» Modern Slavery: servitude, forced labour and exploitation.

Abusers will employ various techniques to engage with their victims; these may include for example: overt attention, verbal seduction (flattery and/or ego stroking), gift-giving and secrecy, as well as threats. They will often claim to have a *special association* with the victim which requires their absolute trust and secrecy – this can make disclosure highly challenging and sensitive.

SnapShot on ... **Mate crime**

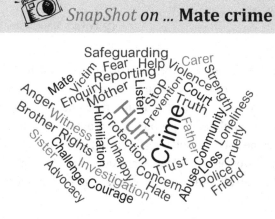

There is no statutory definition of *mate crime* in UK law; the term is generally understood to refer to the befriending of people who are perceived by the perpetrator/source of harm to be vulnerable for the purposes of exploiting and/or abusing them. This can be strongly associated, but not exclusively, with people with learning difficulties or mental health conditions. The graphic above shows some of the words associated with mate crime.

Mate crime can resonate with cases of domestic abuse, but involves additional complex issues. The perpetrator/source of harm is likely to be perceived by the victim to be a close and trusted friend, carer or family member; they will use this relationship as a means for exploitation.

A person experiencing mate crime can be unaware of the perpetrator's motives, and feel unable to challenge or exert control to change their situation of hurt and abuse.

Features and signs of mate crime

It can be difficult to recognise and intervene in cases of mate crime as it is often a pattern of repeat or worsening abuse which has occurred before any concerns are highlighted. The victim may experience:

» Fear of reporting: the person may not recognise that what is happening is wrong; they may be afraid of the consequences of disclosing.

» Social isolation from their usual social contacts or sudden changes in their social network.

» Lack of support: people who are targeted may often be those who do not meet threshold criteria for a high level of support from statutory agencies.

» Coercion, intimidation or threats from their abuser as a means of control.

» Withdrawal or removal from their usual social routines.

» Unexplained physical injuries.

» Lack of access to their money: bills may not be paid.

» Changes in mood and physical presentation: more aggressive or more withdrawn; weight loss; deterioration in personal appearance.

The perpetrator may expose their victim to one or more of the following forms of abuse:

» financial;

» emotional;

» physical;

» criminal exploitation;

» sexual.

> In many situations mate crime may be examples of Disability Hate Crime and as such should be reported to the Police, with a Safeguarding Adults Concern submitted to the local Safeguarding Adults Team.

The concept and application of a risks and strengths approach in cases of self-neglect is a complex area in social work practice, with many varying facets interwoven together. This chapter has aimed to describe a practical and consistent model basis which can be adopted by practitioners from across a broad spectrum of service areas and agencies involved with people who are currently, or in the future may be, at risk of harm through self-neglect. The *Taking it Further* section below suggests an international range of interesting, thought-provoking and useful reading materials and information resources, which demonstrate that self-neglect is truly a worldwide issue of concern.

Taking it Further

Publications

Aiono, V (2011) A Case Study – Using Structured Dependency to Redress Neglect. *Social Work Now: The Practice Journal of Child, Work & Family*, 48: 33–7.

Agazarian, Y (2004) *Systems-Centered Therapy for Groups*. H. Karnac Books Ltd.

Burnett, J, Dyer, C B, Booker, J G, Flores, D V, Green, C E and Diamond, P M (2014) Community-Based Risk Assessment of Elder Mistreatment and Self-Neglect: Evidence of Construct Validity and Measurement Invariance Across Gender and Ethnicity *Journal of the Society for Social Work and Research*, 5(3): 291–319.

Clement, S et al (2011) Disability Hate Crime and Targeted Violence and Hostility: A Mental Health and Discrimination Perspective. *Journal of Mental Health*, 20(3), 219–25.

Director of Public Prosecutions (DPP) (2013) *Code for Crown Prosecutors*, issued under section 10 of the Prosecution of Offences Act 1985.Dong, X and Simon, M (2016) Prevalence of Elder Self-Neglect in a Chicago Chinese population: The Role of Cognitive Physical and Mental Health. *Geriatrics & Gerontology International*, 16(9): 1051–62.

Jakhar, K, Bhatia, T, Saha, R and Deshpande, S N (2015) A Cross Sectional Study of Prevalence and Correlates of Current and Past Risks in Schizophrenia. *Asian Journal of Psychiatry*, 1436–41.

Rutter, M (1985) Resilience in the Face of Adversity: Protective Factors and Resistence to Psychiatric Disorder. *British Journal of Psychiatry*, 147: 598–611.

Thomas, P (2011) 'Mate Crime': Ridicule, Hostility and Targeted Attacks against Disabled People. *Disability & Society*, 26(1): 107–11.

Woolf, S (1995) The Concept of Resilience. *Australian and New Zealand Journal of Psychiatry*, 29(4): 565–74.

Websites

Crown Prosecution Service (2017) Disability Hate Crime and Other Crimes Against Disabled People – Prosecution Guidance. [online] Available at: www.cps.gov.uk/legal-guidance/disability-hate-crime-and-other-crimes-against-disabled-people-prosecution-guidance (accessed (16 December 2017).

Home Office (2014) Modern Slavery. [online] Available at: www.gov.uk/government/collections/modern-slavery (accessed 16 December 2017).

References

Crown Prosecution Service (2013) *The Code for Crown Prosecutors* (issued by the Director of Public Prosecutions). [online] Available at: www.cps.gov.uk/sites/default/files/documents/publications/code_2013_accessible_english.pdf (accessed 16 May 2017).

Crown Prosecution Service (2014) *Domestic Abuse Guidelines for Prosecutors* (issued by the Director of Public Prosecutions). [online] Available at: www.cps.gov.uk/legal-guidance/domestic-abuse-guidelines-prosecutors (accessed 16 May 2017).

Department of Health (2017) *The Care and Support Statutory Guidance.* [online] Available at: www.gov.uk/government/publications/care-act-statutory-guidance/care-and-support-statutory-guidance (accessed 16 May 2017).

Home Office (2015) Statutory Advice Framework: Controlling or Coercive Behaviour in an Intimate or Family Relationship Statutory Guidance Framework. [online] Available at: https://www.gov.uk/government/publications/statutory-guidance-framework-controlling-or-coercive-behaviour-in-an-intimate-or-family-relationship (accessed 16 May 2017).

Independent (2016, 2 December) Deadly 'Legal Highs' Can Now Be 'Ordered like a Takeaway' Because of Government Ban, Users Say. [online] Available at: www.independent.co.uk/news/homelesshelpline/legal-highs-ban-war-on-drugs-spice-mamba-nps-homeless-helpline-centrepoint-charity-christmas-appeal-a7449536.html (accessed 16 May 2017).

NHS National Patient Safety Agency (2008) *A Risk Matrix for Risk Managers.* [online] Available at: www.npsa.nhs.uk/nrls/improvingpatientsafety/patient-safety-tools-and-guidance/risk-assessment-guides/risk-matrix-for-risk-managers/ (accessed 16 May 2017).

Survivors Manchester (n.d.) Grooming. [online] Available at: www.survivorsmanchester.org.uk/impact/legacy-issues/grooming/ (accessed 31 March 2017).

UK Government (1999) *Youth Justice and Criminal Evidence Act.* [online] Available at: http://www.legislation.gov.uk/ukpga/1999/23/contents (accessed 16 May 2017).

Introduction

This chapter looks at illustrative case scenarios using the risks and strengths assessment model framework and associated example documentation. A descriptive 'volcano effect' graphic (Figures 4.1 and 4.2) is included with each case study as a visual learning tool. These illustrations are designed to reflect the multi-faceted and complex nature of self-neglect in adults, and offer example support planning elements. The analogy of a volcano was created as an aid for representing how key factors of self-neglect interact and can contribute to situations which require the supportive intervention of others, these being:

 » Mental Health;

 » Physical Health;

 » Environment;

 » Exploitation/Abuse;

 » Social Network;

 » Attachment.

Each case study described below contains details of the applicable individual factors of self-neglect and the level of risk posed.

Case study 1: A case of infestation and squalor

Background:

Referral to the local Learning Disability Team has been made by an Environmental Health Officer following complaints received from a neighbour regarding an infestation of rodents in Ms A's property which had extended to their home.

Social circumstances:

Ms A is a 57-year-old female who has diagnosed learning difficulties; she had lived all of her life with her parents in a privately owned property. There was no front garden to the property, a courtyard at the rear and net curtains to all windows

Some years earlier both of Ms A's parents had died; she remained living within her family home and had been supported by her elder sibling with all home/financial management tasks (standing orders set up with the bank for all household bills) until their death. A solicitor was involved with financial management and acted as Ms A's appointee for welfare benefit matters.

Ms A was in regular contact with a community health practitioner who didn't visit the home; their meetings took place at a local café or other community facilities.

Ms A followed a rigid daily routine which included going out into the local community each day and visits to a local care home where her father had lived prior to his death – no changes to her physical presentation were noted (she was known to be eccentric in her dress and presentation).

Ms A had no relationship with her neighbours and did not communicate with them. Following referral to the local Environmental Health Department it was found that:

» There was a pet dog living within the property – using an upstairs room as a toilet (dog did not go outside at all).

» The sole toilet in the property was completely blocked and not functioning.

» The property was infested by rodents, insects, with clutter and squalor.

Mental Capacity Act status:

» Lack of capacity to undertake or complete essential home/financial management tasks.

» Holds capacity to make small daily purchases at a local café and shop.

» Lack of capacity in relation to meeting the care/welfare needs of an animal.

» Lack of capacity to decide where to live.

Presenting Action Areas:

» Risks and strengths assessment and support planning involving Ms A (Tables 4.1 and 4.2)

» Independent advocacy

» Mental Capacity Act (2005) Best Interests decision-making

» Animal safety

» De-infestation and clearing/cleaning/decontamination of the property – requiring temporary accommodation elsewhere for Ms A

» Immediate repairs to the essential utilities at the property

» Appointment of a deputy via the Court of Protection

Table 4.1 Ms A – Risk and Strengths Assessment

SELF-NEGLECT – Risk and Strengths Assessment Model								
Name of Adult at Risk:	Ms A							
Unique Identifier:	Case Example 1							
Completed by:	Chrysalis							
Date completed:	02/01/2017							
KEY FACTOR	DESCRIPTION/PROMPTS	ACTUAL RISKS	Impact	Likelihood	Grading	ACTIONS TO BE TAKEN	TIMESCALE	RESPONSIBLE PERSON/ AGENCY
Mental Health	Diagnosed Mental Health condition, learning difficulties and/or impaired cognition; including Diogenes and/or Noah syndrome. Recent deterioration in mental health state (may include the lack of motivation to meet essential personal care needs, recent loss/bereavement, and/or traumatic event). Involvement with specialist healthcare professional.	Diagnosed learning difficulties. Ongoing involvement with the Anytown Learning Disability Team – regular meetings with a Community Health Practitioner. These meeting always take place in community settings (eg local café). Assessed to lack capacity to manage her home environment and household finances without significant support.	3	5	15	Refer to Anytown Advocacy Service. Complete Safeguarding Support Plan with Ms A, supported by an advocate. Confirm arrangements re: the support Ms A needs re: management of her home environment, finances and health.	Ongoing, Review 1 week.	Social worker with team manager.

SELF-NEGLECT – Risk and Strengths Assessment Model

	Non-concordance with treatment plan and/or prescribed medication regime.	Ms A's brother (now deceased) had arranged *all* household bills to be paid by Direct Debit – a local solicitor is appointee for welfare benefits and executor. Ms A manages small amounts of personal money each week.					
	Lack of or fluctuating mental capacity to make informed decisions in this regard, following assessment in line with the requirements of the Mental Capacity Act (2005).						
	Known pattern of problematic alcohol use/ dependency.						
	Known pattern of illegal substance misuse.						
	Involvement with the Police and/or Probation Service (may include MAPPA).						
Physical Health	Recognised 'Long-term/ Enduring Condition' for which treatment/medicine is prescribed.	No presenting risks in this area at this time.	1	1	1	Refer to GP for health check to be completed.	Ongoing. Review 1 week. Social worker.
	'Long-term/Enduring Condition' which has the potential to reduce life expectancy if not managed.						
	Deterioration in physical health state and/or exacerbation of existing condition.						

SELF-NEGLECT – Risk and Strengths Assessment Model								
KEY FACTOR	DESCRIPTION/PROMPTS	ACTUAL RISKS	Impact	Likelihood	Grading	ACTIONS TO BE TAKEN	TIMESCALE	RESPONSIBLE PERSON/ AGENCY
	Involvement with specialist healthcare professionals. Non-concordance with treatment plan and/or prescribed medication regime.							
Housing	Non-secure tenure – may be assured shorthold or informal arrangement (this can include for example bed and breakfast accommodation and/or 'sofa-surfing'). Not suitable to meet needs – mobility or environmental factors. Inadequate essential amenities (utilities). Refusal to engage with support agencies. Insanitary conditions and/or hoarding (objects and/or animals), which will lead to the involvement of Environmental Health Services and may also include Fire Services.	Privately owned, end of terrace property. Solicitor is appointee for welfare benefits and executor. No front garden to the property, courtyard at the rear with net curtains to all window. Pet dog living within the property – using an upstairs room (dog does not go outside at all). Toilet completely blocked and not functioning. Home infested by mice, clutter and squalor. Health and safety risks to Ms A, her neighbours and the dog. Arrange short-term accommodation for Ms A away from the property while clearance, cleaning and de-infestation are completed.	5	5	25	Refer to RSPCA and Environmental Health for immediate removal of the animal at the property, and treatment of the infestation. Contact the solicitor involved to support repairs to the property. Referral to the Court of Protection for the appointment of a deputy/ deputies to support health, welfare and finance issues. Refer to Anytown Advocacy Service.	Immediate. Review 1 week.	Social worker with team manager.

SELF-NEGLECT – Risk and Strengths Assessment Model

Social Network						Social worker.
Relationships – which may be problematic, hazardous and/or abusive (including alcohol/substance dependencies).	Ms A followed a rigid daily routine which included going out into the local community each day and visits to a local care home where her father had lived prior to his death – she has no individually reliable social network.	1	1	1	Arrange a short-term care home placement close to Ms A's known community in order to promote and maintain her involvement and independence.	
Children and/or other adults at risk living at the property.						
Limited/no reliable social network of family/friends *and/or* risks posed by a carer.						
Known pattern of involvement with the criminal justice system.						
Known pattern of involvement with statutory agencies (including crisis intervention).						
Homelessness.						
Debt with inadequate resources to meet demands.						
Involvement with the Police and/or Probation Service (may include MAPPA).						
Young adults at risk in Transition from Children to Adult Social Care Services.						

SELF-NEGLECT – Risk and Strengths Assessment Model

KEY FACTOR	DESCRIPTION/PROMPTS	ACTUAL RISKS	Impact	Likelihood	Grading	ACTIONS TO BE TAKEN	TIMESCALE	RESPONSIBLE PERSON/ AGENCY
Exploitation/ Abuse	Involvement with statutory agencies regarding allegations of abuse (in line with Safeguarding Adults definition). Known involvement with criminal justice offenders and/or perpetrators of abuse. Low self-esteem/worth 'attention-seeking' behaviours which are potentially hazardous (eg attachment disorders). Changes in usual routines, refusal to discuss the basis or nature of these changes. Deterioration in 'usual' personal presentation; this may include physical signs of assault and/ or withdrawal from engagement/involvement. Involvement with the Police and/or Probation Service (may include MAPPA). Young adults at risk in Transition from Children to Adult Social Care Services.	Ms A is vulnerable to exploitation and abuse; however, at this time there is no evidence that this has occurred. Ms A is at an increased level of self-neglect, which poses risks to both her and others.	4	4	16	Arrange a short-term care home placement close to Ms A's known community in order to promote and maintain her involvement and independence. Complete essential environmental works to the property.		Social worker.

SELF-NEGLECT – Risk and Strengths Assessment Model

Organisational					
Rumours; potential for public concern. Local, short-term media coverage – minimal public concern. Local media coverage – long-term reduction in public confidence. National media coverage – long-term reduction in public confidence. National media coverage, which includes the attention of the local parliamentary representative and a total loss of public confidence. Complaint which may include referral and/or investigation by the Ombudsman. Criteria for a Safeguarding Adults Review may be met. Potential for Litigation; criminal prosecution. Breach(es) in statutory duty MAPPA arrangements.	Potential for adverse local media coverage and public concern regarding the level of self-neglect evidenced and the involvement of statutory services.	3	3	9	Continue to gather relevant information. Ensure all case records are accurate and up to date – documenting all decision-making processes; confirming the involvement of Ms A and her advocate/deputy.	Social worker with team manager.

Outcome Risk Levels are confirmed in the 'Volcano Effect' (Figure 4.1) graphic below.

Figure 4.1 Ms A volcano effect

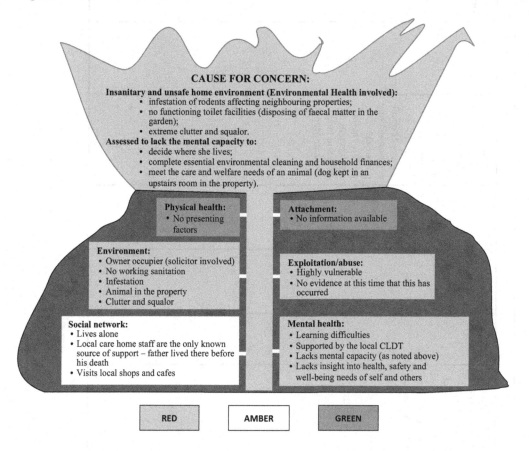

CAUSE FOR CONCERN:
Insanitary and unsafe home environment (Environmental Health involved):
- infestation of rodents affecting neighbouring properties;
- no functioning toilet facilities (disposing of faecal matter in the garden);
- extreme clutter and squalor.

Assessed to lack the mental capacity to:
- decide where she lives;
- complete essential environmental cleaning and household finances;
- meet the care and welfare needs of an animal (dog kept in an upstairs room in the property).

Physical health:
- No presenting factors

Attachment:
- No information available

Environment:
- Owner occupier (solicitor involved)
- No working sanitation
- Infestation
- Animal in the property
- Clutter and squalor

Exploitation/abuse:
- Highly vulnerable
- No evidence at this time that this has occurred

Social network:
- Lives alone
- Local care home staff are the only known source of support – father lived there before his death
- Visits local shops and cafes

Mental health:
- Learning difficulties
- Supported by the local CLDT
- Lacks mental capacity (as noted above)
- Lacks insight into health, safety and well-being needs of self and others

RED   AMBER   GREEN

Table 4.2 Ms A Safeguarding Support Plan (illustrative elements include):

Outcome desired	Action required	Person / Agency responsible	Timescale
Ms A to be supported in maintaining her accommodation and her independence	1. Arrange short-term placement within a registered care home – to include Independent Living Skills Care Plan. 2. Refer to the Court of Protection for the appointment of deputy/deputies to manage Health and Welfare & Finances. 3. Solicitor involved to fund clearing, cleaning and repairs to the property from the monies held on Ms A's behalf. 4. Referral to RSPCA for the care of the dog	Example social worker with community health practitioner	Immediate – date of plan

Outcome desired	Action required	Person / Agency responsible	Timescale
	5. Environmental Health to coordinate the de-infestation of the property 6. Identify potential Supported Living options (eg: assured shorthold tenancy with Support)		
Ms A's involvement and control and co-production of immediate and future care/ support planning and arrangements	1. Referral to Anytown Advocacy Project and Court of Protection.	Example social worker	Immediate – date of plan
Ms A's continued involvement with her local community	1. Arrange short-term placement within/ close to Ms A's home, and arrange plans for her continued visits to local cafes and the care home.	Example social worker with community health practitioner	Review 1 week
Ms A's continued control, with support as required, of her weekly personal finances	1. Contact the solicitor involved to maintain current arrangements for Ms A's access to her weekly personal money.	Example social worker	Immediate
Ms A to have a health check	1. Refer to Ms A's GP and learning disability team consultant for review	Community health practitioner	Review 1 week
Relapse Prevention Plan	Ensure Ms A has access to: • an independent advocate; • accurate and up-to-date information regarding her future options (rights and responsibilities) in line with the Mental Capacity Act (2005) and the Human Rights Act (1998) as applicable; • referral to the Court of Protection.		
Indicators/ triggers for further action	Monitoring of: • Ms A's continued commitment to the short-term care placement arrangements.		
Contingency plan in the event of any further/on-going concerns	A review should be immediately arranged should Ms A withdraw from agreement with current plans, to confirm: • Mental Capacity Act requirements, as appropriate/applicable; • Any other legal implications.		
Review date	**1 week from the date of this Support Plan**		

Case study 2: The threat of eviction and hoarding

Background

Complaints had been made to the local Police Authority by Mr B's neighbours as they were concerned about harassment by local youths. A Police Officer visited Mr B at his home; referral was then made to Adult Social Care.

Social circumstances

Mr B is a 46-year-old male with no diagnosed physical or mental health conditions, who lived alone in a privately rented flat. The property had been found to be an example of extreme hoarding in that all rooms were filled to the ceiling with rotting food, carrier bags/boxes, leaflets for local shops, discarded clothing and other objects – these were not collections of personal items.

Mr B had resided at the property for two years and had had no previous involvement with Adult Social Services. The landlord was threatening to evict him as he alleged that Mr B had damaged his property and broken the terms of his tenancy – he had applied to the local court for an eviction order. Mr B had experienced *low-level harassment* from local youths; this had consisted of name-calling

Mr B had formerly been employed in a customer service position, but had been sacked due to deterioration in his personal appearance and hygiene – he was in receipt of welfare benefits due to unemployment. Mr B had infrequent contact with family members and had no visitors to his home.

Mr B showed and described no personal attachment to the objects in his flat, and recognised that he was unable to access the kitchen, bathroom/toilet or sleeping facilities due to the amount of accumulated clutter.

Mental Capacity Act status

Mr B had the mental capacity to manage all aspects of his life.

Presenting Action Areas:

» Risks and Strengths Assessment & Support Planning involving Mr B (Tables 4:3 and 4:4)

» Independent advocacy

» Referral to the Environmental Health Department

» Further consideration of Mr B's executive mental capacity

» De-infestation and clearing/cleaning/decontamination of the property

» Secure alternative housing (subject to the eviction order being granted)

Table 4.3 Mr B – Risk and Strengths Assessment

SELF-NEGLECT – Risk and Strengths Assessment Model								
Name of Adult at Risk:	Mr B							
Unique Identifier:	Case Example 2							
Completed by:	Chrysalis							
Date completed:	02/01/2017							
KEY FACTOR	**DESCRIPTION/ PROMPTS**	**ACTUAL RISKS**	**Impact**	**Likelihood**	**Grading**	**ACTIONS TO BE TAKEN**	**TIMESCALE**	**RESPONSIBLE PERSON/ AGENCY**
Mental Health	Diagnosed Mental Health condition, learning difficulties and/or impaired cognition; including Diogenes and/or Noah syndrome. Recent deterioration in mental health state (may include the lack of motivation to meet essential personal care needs, recent loss/bereavement, and/or traumatic event).	None known. Previous involvement with the local Police Authority due to complaints raised by his neighbours due to his personal presentation (unkempt and odorous) and concerns regarding low-level harassment by local youths.	1	1	1	None at this time.	Review in 1 week.	Example social worker.

SELF-NEGLECT – Risk and Strengths Assessment Model

Involvement with specialist healthcare professionals.						
Non-concordance with treatment plan and/or prescribed medication regime.						
Lack of or fluctuating mental capacity to make informed decisions in this regard, following assessment in line with the requirements of the Mental Capacity Act (2005).						
Known pattern of problematic alcohol use/dependency.						
Known pattern of illegal substance misuse.						
Involvement with the Police and/or Probation Service (may include MAPPA).						

SELF-NEGLECT – Risk and Strengths Assessment Model

KEY FACTOR	DESCRIPTION/ PROMPTS	ACTUAL RISKS	Impact	Likelihood	Grading	ACTIONS TO BE TAKEN	TIMESCALE	RESPONSIBLE PERSON/ AGENCY
Physical Health	Recognised 'Long-term/Enduring Condition' for which treatment/medicine is prescribed	No physical illness; Mr B is not registered with a GP.	2	4	8	Support Mr B to register with a local surgery.	Review in 1 week.	Example social worker.
	'Long-term/Enduring Condition' which has the potential to reduce life expectancy if not managed.							
	Deterioration in physical health state and/or exacerbation of existing condition.							
	Involvement with specialist healthcare professionals.							
	Non-concordance with treatment plan and/or prescribed medication regime.							

SELF-NEGLECT – Risk and Strengths Assessment Model

Housing			5	5	25		Review in 1 week.	Example social worker with environmental health officers.
	Non-secure tenure – may be assured shorthold or informal arrangement (this can include for example bed and breakfast accommodation and/or 'sofa-surfing'). Not suitable to meet needs – mobility or environmental factors. Inadequate essential amenities (utilities). Refusal to engage with support agencies. Insanitary conditions and/or hoarding (objects and/or animals), which will lead to the involvement of Environmental Health Services and may also include Fire Services.	Threat of eviction – currently an application has been made to the Court. Mr B's home environment is extremely cluttered to the extent that he is unable to access essential amenities. Environmental Health to be actively involved due to the insanitary conditions and threat to the health, safety and well-being of both Mr B and his neighbours.				Ongoing work to support Mr B to engage with and work with Officers from the Environmental Health Department. Referral to the Fire Service for home safety assessment. Arrangement for clearing of the property to commence with Mr B. Skips to be ordered, and a cleaning company to be engaged with Mr B's support.		

SELF-NEGLECT – Risk and Strengths Assessment Model								
KEY FACTOR	**DESCRIPTION/ PROMPTS**	**ACTUAL RISKS**	**Impact**	**Likelihood**	**Grading**	**ACTIONS TO BE TAKEN**	**TIMESCALE**	**RESPONSIBLE PERSON/ AGENCY**
Social Network	Relationships – which may be problematic, hazardous and/or abusive (including alcohol/substance dependencies). Children and/or other adults at risk living at the property. Limited/no reliable social network of family/friends *and/or* risks posed by a carer. Known pattern of involvement with the criminal justice system. Known pattern of involvement with statutory agencies (including crisis intervention). Homelessness. Debt with inadequate resources to meet demands.	Mr B was a formerly employed and manages his own monies – he was in receipt welfare benefits. Limited contact with immediate family. No other social relationships. Police previously involved due to complaints from neighbours.	3	4	12	Ongoing work with Mr B to establish a trusting relationship and address current needs.	Review in 1 week.	Example social worker with team manager.

SELF-NEGLECT – Risk and Strengths Assessment Model							
	Involvement with the Police and/or Probation Service (may include MAPPA). Young adults at risk in Transition from Children to Adult Social Care Services.						Example social worker with team manager.
						Review in 1 week.	
					Ongoing work with Mr B to establish a trusting relationship and address current needs.		
				9			
Exploitation/ Abuse	Involvement with statutory agencies regarding allegations of abuse (in line with Safeguarding Adults definition). Known involvement with criminal justice offenders and/or perpetrators of abuse. Low self-esteem/ worth. 'Attention-seeking' behaviours which are potentially hazardous (eg attachment disorders). Changes in usual routines, refusal to discuss the basis or nature of these changes.	Police previously involved due to complaints from neighbours. Mr B had experienced 'low-level harassment' from local youths; this had consisted of 'name-calling'.	3	3			

SELF-NEGLECT – Risk and Strengths Assessment Model

KEY FACTOR	DESCRIPTION/ PROMPTS	ACTUAL RISKS	Impact	Likelihood	Grading	ACTIONS TO BE TAKEN	TIMESCALE	RESPONSIBLE PERSON/ AGENCY
	Deterioration in 'usual' personal presentation; this may include physical signs of assault and/or withdrawal from engagement/ involvement. Involvement with the Police and/or Probation Service (may include MAPPA). Young adults at risk in Transition from Children to Adult Social Care Services.							
Organisational	Rumours; potential for public concern. Local, short-term media coverage – minimal public concern. Local media-coverage – long-term reduction in public confidence. National media coverage – long-term reduction in public confidence.	Potential for adverse local media attention.	2	2	4	Continue to gather relevant information. Ensure all case records are accurate and up to date – documenting all decision-making processes; confirming the involvement of Mr B.	Review in 1 week.	Example social worker with team manager.

SELF-NEGLECT – Risk and Strengths Assessment Model

National media coverage which includes the attention of the local parliamentary representative and a total loss of public confidence.						
Complaint which may include referral and/or investigation by the Ombudsman.						
Criteria for a Safeguarding Adults Review may be met.						
Potential for Litigation; criminal prosecution.						
Breach(es) in statutory duty						
MAPPA arrangement.						

Outcome Risk Levels are confirmed in the following 'Volcano Effect' graphic representation (Figure 4.2)

Figure 4.2 Volcano effect for Mr B

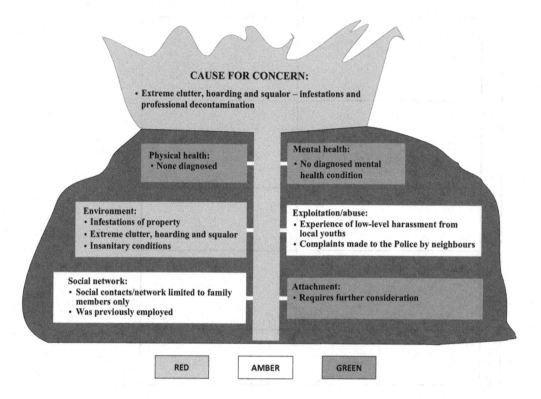

Table 4.4 Mr B – Safeguarding Support Plan (illustrative elements include)

Outcome desired	Action required	Person/ Agency responsible	Timescale
Mr B to be supported in maintaining independence and his rights to privacy and family life in line with both the Mental Capacity Act (2005) and the Human Rights Act (1998), while ensuring that the agencies involved have effectively discharged their statutory duties.	1. Formal completion of assessment of Mr B's mental capacity and executive functioning. 2. Confirmation of his right to make unwise decisions as applicable.	Mental health psychiatrist with community psychiatric nurse.	Immediate – date of plan.

Outcome desired	Action required	Person/ Agency responsible	Timescale
Mr B's involvement and control and co-production of immediate and future care/support planning and arrangements. Encourage Mr B to agree to referral to Anytown Advocacy Project.	1. Develop relationship with Mr B to establish trust. 2. Encourage clearing of priority areas within the flat: a. Kitchen – rotten foods b. Bathroom and toilet 3. Act as liaison between Mr B and Environmental Health. 4. Arrange for a skip to be delivered. 5. Confirm planning and actions with team manager via Supervision Session.	Example social care worker with environmental health officer.	Immediate – date of plan.
Mr B to be registered with a GP.	1. Support Mr B to access health care services.	Example social care worker.	Review 1 week.
Relapse Prevention Plan	Encourage Mr B to access local Independent Advocacy services. Continued interventions undertaken by Example Social Worker to establish a relationship of trust and cooperation. With Mr B's continued consent, pursue joint working with Environmental Health and the Landlord to achieve his continued tenancy.		
Indicators/triggers for further action	Monitoring of Mr B's continued involvement in support planning.		
Contingency plan in the event of any further/on-going concerns	A review should be arranged with all applicable individuals and agencies; this will dictate future support planning and any other applicable legal implications.		
Review date	**2 weeks from the date of this Support Plan**		

Summary

In summary, Case Study 1, as detailed above, contains elements relating to the Mental Capacity Act (2005) and the Care Act (2014). It also highlights the role of carers as a source of strength which mitigated risks associated with self-neglecting behaviors and potential Safeguarding Adults concerns. Ms A was able to manage small amounts of money to make daily purchases and visit her local cafe; however, she lacked the capacity to manage household bills and larger expenditure. Ms A's parents and then her brother had held responsibility for prompting her to complete essential personal and environmental hygiene tasks, also ensuring that all household bills were paid while they were alive. These resources were *strengths* in Ms A's life which, for a time, mitigated known risks to her health, safety and well-being. The loss of these *strengths* was pivotal in Ms A's severe deterioration in personal and environmental circumstances. The Mental Capacity Act (2005) required that Ms A be supported by an Independent Mental Capacity Advocate (IMCA).

In contrast, Case Study 2 differs in many aspects. Mr B had the mental capacity to live his life as he chose, and had no recognised or diagnosed disability, impairment or illness. This may have been a case of unrecognised Diogenes syndrome, in which Mr B showed signs of egosyntonic thinking in that he felt no concern or anxiety with his self-image and chosen lifestyle. The legal frameworks applicable in this case example primarily concerned matters of public health and safety; however, with retrospective review, responsibilities enshrined within the Care Act (2014) may also now hold relevance with the right of access to independent advocacy in this type of circumstance.

Practice matters ...

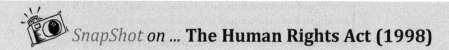

SnapShot on ... The Human Rights Act (1998)

To deny people their human rights is to challenge their very humanity

Nelson Mandela (1918–2015)

The Human Rights Act (1998) placed a legal duty on *public bodies* to work compatibly with the European Convention on Human Rights (1950). This includes the duty to intervene proportionately to protect the rights of citizens. The Human Rights Act (1998) comprises 16 Articles (basic rights) which are all derived from the European Convention.

The following Articles are considered to be of particular relevance in respect of Safeguarding those people who may be at risk of abuse or neglect (further information is available from the Equality and Human Rights Commission at www. equalityhumanrights.com):

ARTICLE 2 Right to life

Everyone's *right to life* must be protected by law. There are only extremely limited circumstances where it is legally acceptable for the State to use force against a person that results in their death; for example, a police officer can use reasonable force to defend themselves or to protect other people.

ARTICLE 3 Prohibition of torture

Everyone has the absolute *right to be free of torture* or to not be subjected to treatment or punishment that is inhuman and/or degrading

ARTICLE 4 Right to liberty and security

Everyone has the *right not to be deprived of their liberty*, except in limited cases specified within the Article, for example where they are suspected or convicted of committing a crime, and provided there is a proper legal basis in UK law for their arrest or detention.

ARTICLE 6 Right to a fair trial

Everyone has the *right to a fair and public hearing*, within a reasonable period of time. This applies to both criminal charges being brought, and in cases concerning civil rights and obligations. According to the law a person who is charged with an offence is presumed innocent until proven guilty, and must also be guaranteed certain minimum rights in relation to the conduct of the criminal investigation and trial.

ARTICLE 8 Right to respect for private and family life

Everyone has the *right to respect for their private and family life*, their home and their correspondence. This right can be only be restricted in specified circumstances

ARTICLE 14 Prohibition of discrimination

In the application of all other convention rights, people have the *right to not be treated differently* because of their race, religion, gender, political views or any other protected characteristics unless there is an 'objective justification' for the difference.

(Human Rights, *Human Lives: A Guide to the Human Rights Act for Public Authorities*)

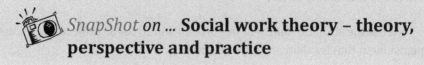

SnapShot on ... **Social work theory – theory, perspective and practice**

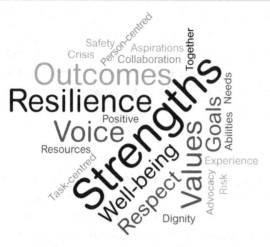

This *SnapShot...* provides an overview of key Social Work Theory, perspective and practice which the authors believe have been proven to be effective when supporting adults who may be at risk.

The approaches described below in Table 4.5 are not exhaustive; practitioners should always use their own professional judgement and their agency/organisation policies and procedures.

Table 4.5 Brief overview of social work theories in self-neglect

Theory (brief overview)	Positives	Constraints
Task-centred approach: » Collaboration between the practitioner and person using the service » Mutually agreed contract » Explicit timescale » Actions are guided by the person using the service, their beliefs about themselves and their world	» Clear and straight-forward process of engagement, planning and conclusion » Concise timeframe, which can assist in maintaining focus upon the issues » Strengths and resilience approach » Well supported by research	» Risk of 'over-simplifying' issues » Some people may be too overwhelmed by their personal circumstances and lack the strength and energy to address them » Not effective if the person does not accept the need for the agency to be involved

Crisis intervention:		

» Brief intervention
 	
» Deals with immediate issues rather than longer-term problems
 	
» Can reawaken unresolved issues from the past and offer an opportunity to address 'non-adjustment' to past events
 	
» Assumes that we live in a 'steady state' and are able to manage change
	» Time-limited and task focused
	
	» Can incorporate other theories, eg:
	  • solution-focused
	  • cognitive behavioural
	
	» Can support the person to navigate major events or life transitions
		» May not appropriately support a person who experiences a continuum of crises
		
		» Does not address societal factors such as social isolation, social exclusion, deprivation or poverty

Person-centred approach:		

» Based upon the work of Carl Rogers
 	
» Uses the principles to support the working relationship between the person using the service and the practitioner:
  • everyone has the ability to grow and develop
  • empathy
  • unconditional regard
  • congruence
  • non-directive
	» Re-enforces dignity and the worth of all citizens
	
	» Enables the person to have their own goals and aspirations
	
	» Focus upon building equitable and meaningful working relationships
	
	» Values all forms of life experience
		» Difficult to apply if the person lacks the motivation to engage
		
		» The focus is upon individual change rather than societal factors
		
		» The expressed goals and aspirations of the person may not be a priority or 'on the agenda' of mainstream society

Recovery model:		
» Focus is upon 'recovery' and not illness; used within mental health services. » The key objective is for the person to gain/regain a sense of control and worth, and does not necessarily mean being 'symptom free' » Recognises the unique strengths of the person » Does not define a person by a label or diagnosis	» Gives control to the person » The person is viewed as the expert in their own situation	» Currently this model is used predominantly within mental health services; its broader use has not been fully explored, utilised and implemented

Narrative approach:		
» Gives the person the opportunity to tell their own story, and in the process of doing so, define their own identity » The person is encouraged and enabled to describe their life in their own words	» Can support the person to make sense of change and adjust to their new circumstances or situation	» The person or their family/supporters may not see the value in this approach and may focus upon seeking a 'solution'

This chapter has given summary examples of how a practice-based risks and strengths assessment model can be used to aid consistency in work with people who self neglect. The aim is to achieve positive and effective person-centred outcomes in the context of a range of legislative requirements and social work theory.

The *Taking it Further* section below is designed to prompt further discussion and debate in this highly complex and challenging area of work.

Taking it Further

Publications

Alcock, R (2014) Ian's Story: His Right to Self-determination. *Ethics and Social Welfare*, 8(1): 77–85.

Andersen, E, Raffin-Bouchal, S and Marcy-Edwards, D (2013) 'Do They Think I Am a Pack Rat?' *Journal of Elder Abuse & Neglect*, 25: 438–52.

Dong, X, Simon, M A and Evans, D (2012) The Prevalence of Elder Self-Neglect in a Community-Dwelling population: Hoarding, Hygiene, and Environmental Hazards. *Journal of Aging and Health*, 24(3): 507–24.

Dong, X, Simon, M A, Mosqueda, L and Evans, D (2013) Elder Self-Neglect is Associated with Increased Risk for Elder Abuse in a Community-Dwelling Population: Findings from the Chicago Health and Aging Project. *Journal of Aging and Health*, 25(1): 80–96.

Musson, P (2017) *Making Sense of Theory and its Application to Social Work Practice*. St Albans: Critical Publishing.

Websites

The Equality and Human Rights Commission. [online] Available at www.equalityhumanrights.com/sites/default/files/human_rights_human_lives_a_guide_for_public_authorities.pdf (accessed 18 December 2017).

Introduction

This chapter gives an overview of the Care Act (2014) 'well-being' principle and considers how this interacts and focuses social work practice in cases of self-neglect and safeguarding adults interventions. The *SnapShots* included in this chapter are:

» balancing attitudes and values in person-centred safeguarding;

» the Care Act (2014) and supporting carers;

» a person in a position of trust.

The Care Act (2014) was implemented in England from April 2015; this brought together multiple pieces of legislation which had developed over previous years. This process consolidated the roles, duties and responsibilities placed upon health, social care and partner agencies, including Safeguarding Adults functions. Key aspects of this legislation include:

» the promotion of 'well-being';

» neglect as a factor in Safeguarding Adults;

» placing Safeguarding Adults Boards (SAB) on a statutory footing.

Chapter 1 of the Care Act (2014) addresses the definition of 'well-being' and requires promotion of this concept (Department of Health, 2015). This requirement places the individual at the centre of all interventions undertaken by health and social care agencies and services, in effect 'person-centered' care and support evidenced in practice. A detail of the Care Act (2014) definition of 'well-being' and its relevance to health and social care assessment processes is discussed below.

Chapter 14 of the Care Act (2014) includes details of the duties and responsibilities placed upon local authorities and health trusts in England in relation to Safeguarding Adults. These duties include the protection of adults at risk from abuse and neglect, and also relate to those who are vulnerable due to reliance upon alcohol and drug abuse.

Six principles in Safeguarding Adults

The six principles outlined within the Care Act (2014) apply to all care and support providers, as well as other settings that offer or supply services to adults whose circumstances may put them at risk. These principles are intended to focus and guide all practice interventions:

Empowerment

Supporting and encouraging people to make their own *informed* decisions.

Prevention

It is better to take action before abuse or neglect occur.

Proportionality

The least intrusive response appropriate to the risk presented.

Protection

Support and representation to those in greatest need.

Partnership

Local solutions through services working with their communities. Communities have a part to play in preventing, detecting and reporting abuse and neglect.

Accountability

Accountability and transparency in delivering Safeguarding.

Practice matters ...

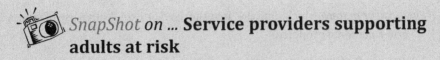

SnapShot on ... Service providers supporting adults at risk

Safeguarding duties apply to an adult (18 years of age and older) who meet the following criteria:

Figure 5.1 Safeguarding Adults' duties

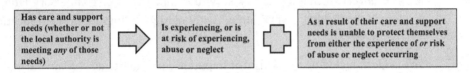

Where abuse or neglect is suspected all agencies involved should aim to intervene in a manner which is:

» *Prompt*: in situations where there is any doubt about the immediate safety and well-being of the adult at risk.

» *Sensitive*: to the person's needs and wishes, and as appropriate, those of their carer/representative.

» *Effective*: in providing or negotiating solutions which are person-centred, as simple and practical as possible, and aim to mitigate the risk of abuse re-occurring.

» *Balanced*: staff must exercise their responsibilities and duties appropriately and proportionately, avoiding unwanted interventions into people's lives.

» *Aware*: does not discriminate against a person because of their race, gender, age, ethnicity, disability, gender identity, sexual orientation or religion.

» *Consider*: signs of abuse or neglect

The information detailed above is a set of brief prompts, which are neither exclusive nor exhaustive practice directions.

An overview of categories of abuse

Physical: including hitting, slapping, biting, squeezing/pinching, restraint or restrictions in movement, pushing or other physical punishment.

Domestic violence or abuse: including coercive and/or controlling behaviours, threatening, assault, social isolation.

Psychological or emotional: including bullying, humiliation, coercion/control, social isolation, removal of required care/support, threats.

Sexual: including touching, penetration, photography, or exploitation to which the person does not or is unable to consent.

Financial or material: including the unauthorised or exploitative use of money or other personal property.

Neglect or act of omission: including the withholding of care and support, ignoring important personal characteristics/wishes.

Organisational: including the failure to ensure that privacy, dignity and respect are shown to the individual and maintained.

Modern slavery: including slavery, servitude and forced or compulsory labour; human trafficking, exploitation; withholding of important identification documents.

Self-neglect: including the refusal or impotence to undertake or complete essential personal and/or environmental health and safety tasks, problematic hoarding of objects and/or animals.

Discrimination: including harassment (assault and/or verbal insults), the withholding of care, ignoring personal needs or wishes on the basis of age, gender, race, religion, ethnicity, disability, sexual orientation or gender identity.

Stop, think, remember ...

» 'Categories of abuse' are a simple guide and not a checklist. Abuse and neglect can take many forms in relation to the individual and at times complex lives people live.

» Patterns of abuse vary; serial abuse, grooming, long-term abuse and opportunistic or 'one-off' events.

» Abuse should always be considered in relation to the individual adult at risk's circumstances and wishes, as well as the impact upon that person's life.

» *All* information, actions and rationale for decisions *must* be recorded and reported accurately.

» The adult at risk and the person raising the concern should be kept informed of the 'next steps'; if this is that, for example, no further action is to be taken or a Section 42 Enquiry is to commence.

These legislative requirements guide and structure approaches to the support of adults who self-neglect or are at risk of self-neglect. As noted previously, there is limited empirical evidence collated in relation to the form and prevalence of self-neg-lect in younger adults; this publication suggests that a key action to address this pau-city of information should include the adoption of a robust, concise and consistently applied risks and strengths model of assessment and planning, to grow knowledge and enable further developments. The two case studies described in Chapter 4 from a practitioner's perspective demonstrate the diverse and atypical presentations which are associated with self-neglect in adults.

The 'well-being' principle

The main components of the 'well-being' principle are detailed within the Act and supporting statutory guidance, and are summarised in Figure 5.2. These factors should guide the assessment of need and co-production of an appropriate support plan with the individual in need.

Figure 5.2 The well-being principle

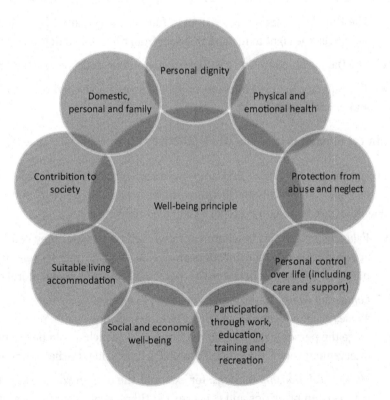

Ascertaining an individual's views and wishes is of equal importance in Safeguarding Adults work, as with all other aspects of assessment and interventions. It is of critical importance in cases of self-neglect, as with all other situations, to assess and confirm the individual's mental capacity to make choices and decisions (as defined within Section 2 (1) of the Mental Capacity Act 2005).

SnapShot on ... **Balancing attitudes and values in person-centred Safeguarding**

Everyone is an individual with their own unique values, attitudes, beliefs and preferences. To achieve an approach to Safeguarding that is 'person-centred', all of those involved need to recognise individuality and diversity, while consulting with and involving the adult at risk at all stages of their safeguarding journey.

Key legal and governance frameworks

» The Care Act (2014) makes it the duty of local authorities to make enquiries if someone is being *or* is at risk of being abused or neglected in their area.

» The Mental Capacity Act (2005) aims to protect and empower people to make informed decisions with or without support. Enforces the requirement for robust assessment of a person's capacity which is issue and time-specific.

» The Human Rights Act (1998) gives fundamental rights to people who live in the UK, eg the right to life and freedom from torture and degrading treatment.

» The Data Protection Act (1998) regulates and protects personal information.

» The Equality Act (2010) protects people from discrimination in the workplace and in wider society.

Ethical dilemmas in social work practice

Ethical dilemmas (Figure 5.3) are woven through social work practice and can, at times, cause uncertainty for the practitioner involved in a case of self-neglect. These dilemmas can be roughly categorised in the following ways:

» *Value dilemmas*: this is where your own personal values may conflict with the action you need to take in your professional role. The authors refer to this as the potential for tension between the 'personal and professional moral compass'.

» *Competing values:* for example, you may be working with a person who regularly abuses drugs and alcohol and this affects their mental health. You have to acknowledge the person's right to self-determination (which would be the basis for not intervening) versus the value of protecting human life (the basis for intervention).

» *Multiple relationship tensions:* for example, the person you are supporting may have certain priorities and concerns *but* there may be parents/carers/spouses in this person's life who view the situation differently and have conflicting concerns. Who do you owe the primary obligation to? The answer should always, of course, be to the adult at risk, but this is not always straightforward particularly in circumstances where the adult at risk is reliant upon the other person to offer and provide care and support.

Figure 5.3 Ethical dilemmas:

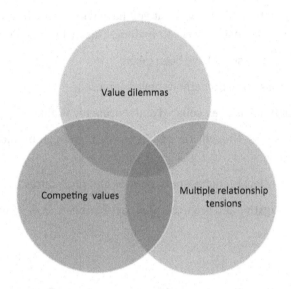

Case example: Family dynamics

An older person who has been self-neglecting and wants to remain living within their own home. Family members want them to move to a registered care home.

A question of rights, and whose problem is this? How would you approach this scenario?

Case example: Potential financial abuse

Mary is a younger adult with whom you have been working for several months; she has complex learning disabilities and impaired cognition and at times her behaviours can be extremely challenging. Mary is supported by her family who are friendly and appear to do a lot for her in very difficult circumstances. Recently Mary has told you that her mother has been taking money from her and has hit her on one occasion. You know that this situation should be reported, but on the other hand you really like Mary's mother and are aware that the family operate under a great deal of stress and pressure. You have the dilemma of wanting to cause the least amount of harm to the family as a whole, while legally you are required to act appropriately to safeguard Mary.

How do you manage the balance of your legal obligations and support with this family?

Defensible *not* defensive decision-making

It is essential that all involvement you have with an adult at risk is based upon and supported by defensible decision-making. This includes assurance that:

» all reasonable steps have been taken;

» reliable assessment methods have been used;

» information has been collated and thoroughly evaluated;

» decisions are 'thought through', recorded, and communicated accurately and effectively;

» applicable legal requirements, policies and procedures have been followed;

» an investigative and proactive approach has been adopted with all interventions.

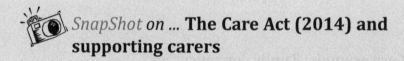

SnapShot on ... The Care Act (2014) and supporting carers

Chapter 14 of the *Care and Support Statutory Guidance* (updated 24 February 2017) contains the following description of duties held by the local authority in relation to 'carers', under the requirements of the Care Act (2014):

14.45 Circumstances in which a carer (for example, a family member or friend) could be involved in a situation that may require a safeguarding response include:

• a carer may witness or speak up about abuse or neglect;

• a carer may experience intentional or unintentional harm from the adult they are trying to support or from professionals and organisations they are in contact with;

• a carer may unintentionally or intentionally harm or neglect the adult they support on their own or with others.

14.46 Assessment of both the carer and the adult they care for must include consideration of the well-being of both people. Section 1 of the Care Act includes protection from abuse and neglect as part of the definition of well-being. As such, a needs or carer's assessment is an important opportunity to explore the individuals' circumstances and consider whether it would be possible to provide information, or support that prevents abuse or neglect from occurring, for example, by providing training to the carer about the condition that the adult they care for has or to support them to care more safely. Where that is necessary the local authority should make arrangements for providing it.

14.47 If a carer speaks up about abuse or neglect, it is essential that they are listened to and that where appropriate a safeguarding enquiry is undertaken and other agencies are involved as appropriate.

14.48 If a carer experiences intentional or unintentional harm from the adult they are supporting, or if a carer unintentionally or intentionally harms or neglects the adult they support, consideration should be given to: whether, as part of the assessment and support planning process for the carer and, or, the adult they care for, support can be provided that removes or mitigates the risk of abuse.

For example, the provision of training or information or other support that minimises the stress experienced by the carer. In some circumstances the carer may need to have independent representation or advocacy; in others, a carer may benefit from having such support if they are under great stress or similar, whether other agencies should be involved; in some circumstances where a criminal offence is suspected this will include alerting the police, or in others the primary healthcare services may need to be involved in monitoring.

14.49 Other key considerations in relation to carers should include:

- involving carers in safeguarding enquiries relating to the adult they care for, as appropriate;

- whether or not joint assessment is appropriate in each individual circumstance;

- the risk factors that may increase the likelihood of abuse or neglect occurring;

- whether a change in circumstance changes the risk of abuse or neglect occurring.

14.50 A change in circumstance should also trigger the review of the care and support plan and/or support plan. Further information about these considerations can be found in an Association of Directors of Adult Social Services (ADASS) paper on carers and safeguarding.

Case example: Carers assessment and support planning

Mrs D lives with her husband, B.

B has a long-term brain injury which affects his mood, behaviour and his ability to manage close family relationships. This has often led to him shouting and hitting out at his wife, who is also his main informal carer. Mrs D told a professional who was involved in supporting her that she was becoming increasingly frightened by B's physical and verbal outbursts and at times feared for her personal safety.

Other family members were unaware of the extent of the harm and that Mrs D was exhausted and considering leaving the situation. The local authority became involved.

The situation presented significant personal risk to Mrs D but there was also a risk of fragmenting relationships if the local authority staff were not sensitive to the needs of the whole family. The practitioner, under supervision from her social work manager, invested time in meeting with Mrs D to explore her preferences around managing her safety and how information about the situation would be communicated with the wider family and with B.

This presented dilemmas around balancing the local authority's duty of care towards Mrs D with her wishes to remain in the situation with B. Placing emphasis on the latter inevitably meant that Mrs D would not be entirely free from the risk of harm but allowed the practitioner to explore help and support options which would enable Mrs D to manage and sustain her safety at a level which was acceptable to her.

The practitioner received regular supervision to allow time to reflect on the support being offered and to ensure that it was 'person-centred'. The outcome for Mrs D was that she was able to continue to care for B by working in partnership with the local authority. The practitioner offered advice about how to safely access help in an emergency and helped her to develop strategies to manage her own safety – this included staff building rapport with B, building on his strengths and desire to participate in social activities outside the family home. The effect of this was that some of the trigger points of him being at home with his wife for sustained periods during the day were reduced because he was there less frequently.

Mrs D also had a number of pre-existing support avenues, including counselling and a good relationship with her son and her friends.

The situation will be reviewed regularly with Mrs D but for the time being she feels much more able to manage.

How do you ensure that you safely adopt a positive risk-taking approach in your practice?

SnapShot on ... **A person in a position of trust**

Simple definition:

A person who works with adults at risk of abuse or neglect on a paid, unpaid or voluntary basis.

The Care Act (2014), and supporting Statutory Guidance (Chapter 14), places the following responsibilities on local authorities (Safeguarding Adults Boards – SAB) and employers of people who work with adults at risk of abuse or neglect on a paid, unpaid or voluntary basis. These responsibilities are quoted directly from the Statutory Guidance and contain the relevant paragraph numbers to support the reader to search efficiently for further information:

a) *14.121:* Safeguarding adults boards need to establish and agree a framework and process for how allegations against people working with adults with care and support needs (for example, those in positions of trust) should be notified and responded to. Whilst the focus of Safeguarding Adults work is to safeguard one or more identified adults with care and support needs, there are occasions when incidents are reported that do not involve an adult at risk, but indicate, nevertheless, that a risk may be posed to adults at risk by a person in a position of trust.

b) *14.122:* Where such concerns are raised about someone who works with adults with care and support needs, it will be necessary for the employer or student body or voluntary organisation to assess any potential risk to adults with care and support needs who use their services, and, if necessary, to take action to safeguard those adults.

c) *14.112:* When a complaint or allegation has been made against a member of staff, including people employed by the adult, they should be made aware of their rights under employment legislation and any internal disciplinary procedures.

d) *14.116:* Employers who are also providers or commissioners of care and support not only have a duty to the adult with care and support needs, but also a responsibility to take action in relation to the employee when allegations of abuse are made against them. Employers should ensure that their recruitment and disciplinary procedures are compatible with the responsibility to protect adults at risk of abuse or neglect.

e) *14.117:* With regard to abuse, neglect and misconduct within a professional relationship, codes of professional conduct and/or employment contracts should be followed and should determine the action that can be taken. Robust employment practices, with checkable references and recent Disclosure and Barring

Service (DBS) checks are important. Reports of abuse, neglect and misconduct should be investigated and evidence collected.

f) *14.118:* Where appropriate, employers should report workers to statutory and other bodies responsible for professional regulation, such as the Health Care Professional Council, General Medical Council and the Nursing and Midwifery Council. If someone is removed from their role (paid worker or unpaid volunteer) because the person poses a risk of harm to adults, a referral to the DBS must be made. This applies even if the person leaves their role to avoid a disciplinary hearing following a safeguarding incident and the employer/volunteer organisation feels they would have dismissed the person based on the information they hold

g) *14.119:* The standard of proof for prosecution is 'beyond reasonable doubt'. The standard of proof for internal disciplinary procedures and for discretionary barring consideration by the DBS and the Vetting and Barring Board is usually the civil standard of 'on the balance of probabilities'. This means that when criminal procedures are concluded without action being taken this does not automatically mean that regulatory or disciplinary procedures should cease or not be considered. In any event there is a legal duty to make a safeguarding referral to DBS if a person is dismissed or removed from their role due to harm to a child or a vulnerable adult.

This chapter has given an overview of the responsibilities placed upon practitioners in work with people who are at risk of self-neglect and their carers. It also recognises the challenges and tensions a practitioner can experience in this area of work and raises the concept of a *person in a position of trust.* The *Taking it Further* suggestions below highlight sources of further information and guidance.

Taking it Further

Publications

Cooper, A, Briggs, M, Lawson, J, Hodson, W and Wilson, M (2016) *Making Safeguarding Personal Temperature Check 2016.* Association of Directors of Adult Social Services. [online] Available at: www.adass.org.uk/making-safeguarding-personal-temperature-check-2016 (accessed 18 December 2017).

References

Association of Directors of Adult Social Services (ADASS) (2011) *Carers and Safeguarding Adults – Working Together to Improve Outcomes. The Care and Support Statutory Guidance.*

Introduction

This chapter suggests an approach, developed by the authors, to building sustainable community strength and resilience. This model directly relates to and interfaces with the role of agencies represented on locality Safeguarding Adults Boards (SAB), in addressing self-neglect and the people who are at risk of self-neglect living in their area. The *SnapShot* in this chapter describes a suggested personalised community consolidation model of practice which places the person at the centre of all interventions from the individual through to multi-agency planning and decision-making.

Safeguarding Adults Boards

In 2000, in recognition of the importance of the principle of collaboration, the UK Government published 'No Secrets', a guidance document promoting inter-agency working to safeguard adults. However, reviews of serious cases of abuse highlighted the weaknesses in the 'guidance only' status of multi-agency working to protect adults; this was replaced by the Care Act (2014).

The Care Act 2014 sought to remedy the shortfalls in inter-agency collaboration by placing SABs on a statutory footing. It is the SAB, compiled of senior representatives from relevant professions within the adult care system that, in consultation with the public, instigates a Strategic Safeguarding Plan for each local authority community. The SAB is in situ to act as a multi-agency umbrella collective which fosters good practice in inter-agency safeguarding practice within its respective locality. The SAB's legislative remit enhances its powers and responsibilities to work with communities to prevent abuse, protect adults from harm or neglect and to hold professionals to account for any failings relating to these priorities.

The six main functions of an SAB

The Care Act identifies six main functions of an SAB:

1. The production of a Safeguarding Strategic Plan.

2. Consultation with Healthwatch and the community in the formulation of such a plan.

3. The completion of Safeguarding Adults Reviews (SARs).

4. Provision of an Annual Report detailing performance against its Strategic Plan.

5. Provision of the annual report to the chief executive of the local authority, the Local Policing Board, the chair of the Health and Well-being Board, and the local Healthwatch organisation.

6. Members' duty to supply information to the SAB for the purpose of enabling it to exercise its functions.

These statutory requirements form the basis of a more formal, structured and accountable approach to joint working in safeguarding adults, which has hitherto been absent from adult social care.

Strategic Safeguarding Plan

The SAB is required to formulate a Strategic Safeguarding Plan for its community, which incorporates both national and local priorities for keeping adults safe. In initiating such a plan, the SAB should consider both short-term and long-term objectives for improving safety. To accommodate long-term aims, the Strategic Safeguarding Plan can cover a period of between three to five years; however, the SAB must review and update the plan on an annual basis, and report on activities via an annual report. The Strategic Safeguarding Plan itself must include not only safeguarding priorities but also the actions required to be taken by each member organisation to achieve the intended outcomes. It should in effect include not only its aims but also a 'road map' indicating the steps to reaching its goals.

Objectives of the Strategic Safeguarding Plan must be compiled with the community, creating a sense of duty that the SAB should serve the community in which it exists. Finally, there is a closure of the performance circle by requiring the SAB to report on its progress to senior management in key agencies, and again the community. This subjects the SAB membership agencies and organisations to scrutiny of its work, and installing an incentive to perform positively against its specified objectives as clear evidence of the development of a proactive preventative approach to Safeguarding Adults, including those at risk of self-neglect.

The key principle of prevention in safeguarding is very much evident within the functions of the SAB; delivery of a Strategic Safeguarding Plan necessitates a three-level approach to be taken (Figure 6.1):

1. To identify and tackle local community issues such as harassment, racism, substance misuse, and exploitation of vulnerable adults, to reduce the risk of harm to members of society. In doing so the Board must engage with the community and harness their help to identify and address issues particular to its area.

2. Individual members must singularly and together assess risk of harm at its early stages to work with the individual to manage risk in a way that reduces its escalation to more significant harm.

3. At the point at which an individual requires help in protecting themselves, professionals, under procedures produced by the SAB, should work together to investigate and make the individual safe.

Figure 6.1 The Strategic Safeguarding Plan

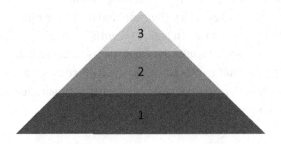

The Safeguarding Adults Board, by addressing Points 1 and 2 above, within the Strategic Plan, should, through thorough planning and preventative work, reduce the number of cases that result in the need for inter-agency protective action in Point 3.

Prevalence and presentations of self-neglect

There is an amplified sense of accountability for agencies to work together. The functions identified for the SAB introduce performance measurement in relation to how well the members carry out collective safeguarding work in the locality to the benefit of the community as a whole; this includes cases of self-neglect in younger adults as well as older people.

Accurate and effective information sharing between agencies, in cases of actual or suspected cases of self-neglect in younger as well as older adults, stand as a key component to the achievement of protection and prevention.

A lack of recognition and research into this area can create a climate within which younger adults at risk of self-neglect can 'fall through the gaps' in traditional service responses and provision.

Key challenges include:

» Lack of empirical information regarding accepted presentations of self-neglect in younger adults and prevalence rates (locally, nationally and internationally).

» A presumption of the mental capacity to choose to live chaotic, insanitary and unsafe lifestyles which can result in self-neglect, harm and sadly, at times, the premature death of a younger adult at risk.

» Unrecognised cases of Diogenes and/or Noah syndrome (with or without hoarding) in younger adults, which may include facets of egosyntonic behaviours and values. In their article Irvine and Nwachukwu (2014) conclude that '*timely diagnosis and respectful management may reduce both acute and chronic physical illness, increase personal and home hygiene and safety, and improve public health outcomes'.*

» The disengagement or non-compliance of a younger adult at risk with services and/or treatment. It is 'best practice' within organisations to have specific guidance in relation to cases of disengagement and non-compliance. This gives staff a structure within which they can maximise the efficiency of their efforts to support those who do not engage well with services, as is evidenced in cases of self-neglect in younger adults. In the majority of cases it is not problematic when a person chooses not to attend or engage with some or all of the services offered to them, but there are occasions in work with younger adults at risk of self-neglect when this can give cause for concern.

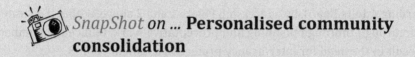

SnapShot on ... **Personalised community consolidation**

Within social approaches to intervention, ranging back to the 1970s, the 'person' has been advocated as central to enquiry, assessment and care/support planning processes.

The translation of this principle into a model for work with people at risk of self-neglect which directly relates to and informs the co-production of support plans, as well as guiding and informing community developments and the commissioning of services to meet known local needs, based upon direct evidence, is described, by the authors, as *personalised community consolidation* (Figure 6.2).

The process of achieving sustainable *personalised community consolidation* begins with the individual adult at risk of self-neglect and their personal issues of concern. As the cohort of people at risk of self-neglect is diverse, the initial information gathering and assessment phases may take extended periods of time, and are fully reliant upon effective multi-agency working and information sharing.

At times of Safeguarding Adults enquiries it may require clear prioritisation of immediate risk of harm or neglect; however, this should not create an artificial barrier to ongoing involvement to firmly establish a trust relationship.

Level 1

Identification and assessment of the specific elements of concern applicable to the adult at risk; these may include, for example, any or all of the following aspects:

» Physical health;

» Mental health;

» Environment (including: lack of security in housing tenure, squalor, hoarding or the welfare of other children/adults at risk, the welfare of animals, fire risk, lack of basic utilities);

» Debt;

» Social network;

» Exploitation – and/or risk;

» Their carer and their right to assessment and support of their own well-being under the Care Act (2014);

» Ethnic identity and risk of exclusion (this can include a lack of common understanding due to the use of jargon and 'professionalised terminology' as well as the need for information to be made readily available in a variety of languages and formats).

Level 2

The availability and accessibility of locally commissioned services and information resources.

» Are they reflective of local needs, with a common culture and value base?

» Are they accessible and accessed by the local community – if not, why not?

» Is there a common understanding and language shared by local agencies – which is also clearly understood by the local community and the individual adult at risk?

» Are services commissioned in effective partnership with the local community based upon *real* 'co-production' principles?

» How does the individual adult at risk engage with the co-production of their support plan?

» Are there unmet needs in relation to the individual adult at risk; how can these be captured and used as an evidence base for future commissioning?

» Are review mechanisms effective in identifying and acting upon needs – both met and unmet?

» Can the individual adult at risk be effectively supported within currently available resources – if not why not?

» Is advocacy required and available?

» Is debt advice required and available?

> » Is housing tenancy related support required and available?

> » Is information readily available in a variety of formats and languages?

Level 3

The use of local needs analysis directs the commissioning of support services.

> » Lessons are learned from all interventions.

> » Evidence of local need is collated and used to develop and sustain community-focused services which effectively inform and support the community as a means to prevent escalation of risk and harm.

Level 4

In keeping the individual adult at risk at the centre of all aspects of local service development, a common culture of community cohesion and consolidation can be achieved and sustained. This dedicated focus, analysis and action, embedded within a commitment to promoting human rights and responsibilities, supports the translation of need to a *preventative approach* to personalise community co-production in support planning based upon local learning.

Figure 6.2 Personalised community consolidation

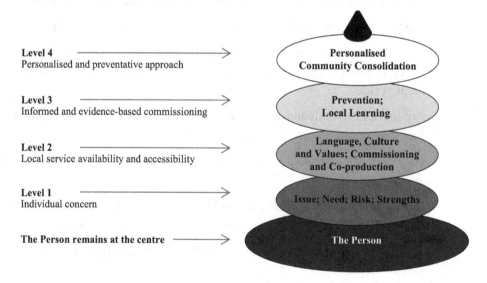

In creating a localised evidence base of self-neglect prevalence rates and presentations, of their own community, a Safeguarding Adults Board will be well placed to create coordinated and effective service development priorities across partner agencies. In adopting a community- and person-centred focus scarce resources can be targeted at key local challenges, as these will differ from area to area, not least because of the significant differences between urban and rural living, and their demography. This chapter has aimed to give emphasis to these ongoing debates, held both nationally and on international platforms.

Taking it Further

Publications

Dong, X, Simon, M and Evans, D (2013). Elder Self-Neglect is Associated with Increased Risk for Elder Abuse in a Community-Dwelling Population: Findings from the Chicago Health and Aging Project. *Journal of Aging and Health*, 25(1): 80–96.

Dong, X and Simon, M (2015) Elder Self-neglect is Associated with an Increased Rate of 30-day Hospital Readmission: Findings from the Chicago Health and Aging Project. *Gerontology*, 61(1): 41–50.

Franzini, L and Dyer, C B (2008) Healthcare Costs and Utilization of Vulnerable Elderly People Reported to Adult Protective Services for Self-Neglect. *Journal of the American Geriatrics Society*, 56(4): 667–76.

Lauder, W, Anderson, I and Barclay, A (2005) Housing and Self-Neglect: The Responses of Health, Social Care and Environmental Health Agencies. *Journal of Interprofessional Care*, 19(4): 317–25.

Reyes-Ortiz, C A, Burnett, J, Flores, D V, Halphen, J M and Dyer, C B (2014) Medical Implications of Elder Abuse: Selfneglect. *Clinics in Geriatric Medicine*, 30(4): 807–23.

References

Department of Health (2017) *Care and Support Statutory Guidance*.

Irvine, J and Nwachukwu, K (2014). Recognizing Diogenes Syndrome: A Case Report. *BMC Research Notes*, 7: 276.

Appendix 1: The Mental Capacity Act (2005)

The Mental Capacity Act (2005) (the Act) applies to individuals aged 16 years and above, who lack the mental capacity to make health, social care or financial decisions. Decisions can include medication, diagnostic tests, allied health professional care, nursing care and social care, including where a person should live, care provided in care homes and domiciliary care. It applies wherever these decisions are made (eg home, hospital, GP, dental practice or care home). If a person lacks mental capacity the Act must be used. The full powers of the Act came into force from October 2007, supported by a comprehensive Code of Practice.

NB: This document should not be regarded as a substitute for the Act itself, or supporting Department of Health publications – it is not intended to be, nor should it be relied upon as legal advice.

Principles of the Mental Capacity Act (2005)

1. Every individual (16+) must be presumed to have capacity unless there is evidence that they do not.

2. A person is *not* to be treated as lacking capacity until *all* practicable steps have been taken to support the person without success.

3. An unwise decision does not mean a person lacks capacity.

4. Any decision or action taken on behalf of a person lacking capacity must be in their best interests.

5. Any decision or taken on behalf of a person lacking capacity should aim to be the least restrictive option possible.

Assessment of Capacity

The two-stage test

» *Stage 1:* Is there an impairment of or disturbance in the functioning of the person's mind or brain? (For example, dementia, brain injury, learning difficulties, confusion due to illness/treatment, drug/alcohol misuse, mental health problem, unconsciousness).

If yes...

» *Stage 2:* Is the impairment or disturbance sufficient that the person lacks the capacity to make that particular decision?

NB: The two-stage test is *time* and *decision* specific.

To have capacity a person must be able to:

» understand information relating to the decision required (including consequences);

» retain the information long enough to make a decision;

» use or 'weigh in the balance' (believe and take into account) the information;

» communicate a decision (in any form which can be reliably recognised).

Failure on any one point means the person lacks capacity – but only at that particular time in relation to that particular decision.

Advance decisions

A statement refusing the future treatment (often called a living will). A person must be 18 and have capacity to make an advance decision. It only comes into force if the person loses capacity. A valid and applicable advance decision must be followed by healthcare staff. To refuse life-sustaining treatment it must be in writing and signed by the person (or by another as directed by them) and witnessed plus also contain a statement that the decision relates to life-sustaining treatment.

Advocacy

A legal right to independent advocacy for some people who lack capacity and for whom important decisions (serious treatment, NHS or local authority, accommodation, care reviews or Adult at Risk procedures) are being made. A legal duty is placed upon NHS bodies and local authorities to use an advocate. The advocate has legal powers, including access to records.

Best interests

If a person fails the test of capacity the best interests checklist must be followed. All the points below must be considered when making a health or social care decision in the person's best interests:

» All relevant circumstances.

» Will the person regain capacity? If so, can the decision wait?

» Consult (as practical and appropriate) others who know the person – friends, carers, relatives, attorneys and deputies.

» Encourage the person to participate in the decision-making process as far as possible.

» Any other factors the person would consider if they could.

» The decision should not be based solely on the person's age, appearance, condition or behaviour.

» For life-sustaining treatment – the decision must be motivated by a desire to bring about the person's death.

The Court of Protection

The Court of Protection was established under the Act to make judgments on disputes concerning the Act. For example, whether a person has capacity on a matter and what is in their best interests. The court will also appoint deputies (see below) to help some people who lack capacity.

Deputies

Deputies are appointed by the Court of Protection to make decisions on behalf of some people who lack capacity. The court decides on the extent and duration of a deputy's powers. Deputies will be appointed where ongoing/serious/disputed decisions (health, social care or financial) need to be made.

Lasting Power of Attorney (LPA)

A person who can appoint someone of their choice (an attorney) to make health and/or social care and/or financial decisions for them should they lack capacity to do so in the future. The person must be 18 and have capacity to make an LPA. The person decides which decisions the attorney can make for them. The LPA only comes into force if the person loses capacity.

The Public Guardian

Responsibilities:

» Provides information and guidance on the Act.

» Monitors and deals with complaints relating to *Lasting Powers of Attorney* and *deputies*.

» Reports to the Court of Protection.

Restraint

The power to restrain a person if:

> » The person lacks capacity to the matter in question and it is in the person's best interests for them to be restrained, and it is reasonable to believe that it is necessary to restrain the person to prevent harm to them and the restraint is a proportionate response to the likelihood of the person suffering harm and the seriousness of that harm.

Research

Before intrusive research (not clinical trials) is carried out, authority to undertake it on people who lack capacity to consent must be approved by:

1. A Research Ethics Committee.

2. People who know the person or someone independent must have been consulted.

3. Other legal Safeguards contained in the Act must have been followed.

Further information

Further information can be sought from the Office of the Public Guardian: 0845 330 2900; www.publicguardian.gov.uk

Appendix 2: The Mental Health Act (1983) – rights, powers and protection

This Appendix simply describes the main sections (detention powers) of the Mental Health Act (1983) (the Act) applicable to people aged 18 years or older – there are other powers (for example, court orders, and those applicable to younger people and children) which are not included. It is designed to give a simple overview of key aspects of the Act.

> **NB: This document should not be regarded as a substitute for the Act itself, or supporting Department of Health publications – it is not intended to be, nor should it be relied upon as legal advice.**

Admission to hospital

There are three main ways in which a person can be admitted to a mental health hospital or other place registered to use the Act; these are:

Informal/Voluntary

A person who has the mental capacity to decide whether to admit themselves to and remain within an in-hospital setting. In this case the person has the right to leave the hospital or discharge themselves from there at any time. They can agree to remain in the hospital or take leave from there for specified periods of time as part of their care plan. The person has the right to consent to or refuse any treatment offered to them. The Mental Health Act Code of Practice (paragraph 2.45) states that informal patients

should be made aware of their legal position and right. Local policies and arrangements about movement around the hospital and its grounds must be clearly explained to the patients concerned. Failure to do so could lead to a patient mistakenly believing that they are not allowed freedom of movement, which could result in an unlawful deprivation of their liberty.

Mental Capacity Act (2005)

This piece of legislation can be used to support a person who lacks the mental capacity to decide for themselves to be admitted to or remain in hospital. Those responsible for admitting the person to hospital complete a test of capacity, regarding this specific issue, under the requirements of the Mental Capacity Act (2005) and confirm their 'Best Interests' decision assessment to authorise the person's admission. This assessment of the person's capacity and the 'Best Interests' decision should be kept under review during the period of inpatient care. In this circumstance the person retains the right to make other decisions unless it is proven that they lack the capacity to make these other decisions by following the Mental Capacity Act (2005) legal requirements. The Mental Capacity Act (2005) applies not only to mental health care treatment but all health care, social care and financial decisions for those assessed as lacking the mental capacity to make issue-specific decisions, at the time the decision needs to be made.

NB: The Mental Capacity Act (2005) also contains the power to deprive a person of their liberty, for example in a hospital setting; this process is called the Deprivation of Liberty Safeguards (DOLS).

Mental Health Act (1983)

The Act can apply whether or not the person has the mental capacity to consent to their admission to hospital based upon the formally assessed severity of their mental disorder; this power also applies to those who need to be detained/prevented from leaving hospital in this circumstance. The criteria for detaining people are given below. The Act does not have age limits for the majority of sections; where this is not the case it is stated.

NB: There are other ways to admit a person to hospital such as under the National Assistance Act 1949, but these are rarely used.

Mental Health Act (1983) Sections – *short-term orders* – no longer than 72 hours in duration

Section 135 (1) Warrant

Purpose

To provide police officers with a power of entry to private premises, for the purposes of removing the person to a place of safety for a mental health assessment or for other arrangements to be made for their treatment or care, based upon assessment completed by an Approved Mental Health Professional (AMHP) and their application to a magistrate for a Section 135 (1) Warrant to be issued.

Legal criteria (these must be met to use the power of this Section)

» There is reasonable cause to suspect a person believed to be suffering from mental disorder has been, or is being, ill-treated, neglected or kept otherwise than under proper control; *or*

» is living alone and is unable to care for themselves.

Duration of Section

Up to 72 hours from when the person is admitted to hospital (or other place of safety).

Any further detention would require a new Section to be completed within 72 hours, ie Section 2 or 3.

Professionals required to comply with and complete this Section

An AMHP applies to a Magistrate for a warrant to be issued; the police officer must be accompanied by an AMHP and a doctor to remove a person for assessment in hospital (*or another place of safety*).

Treatment (what are the treatment powers?)

The person must either consent to treatment or, if they lack capacity, the Mental Capacity Act (2005) may be used to treat them in their best interests.

Leave of absence?

Not applicable – the power provides for short-term detention only.

Duties on staff

The AMHP and all staff involved must inform the person of their legal rights (both verbally and in writing) and take all practicable steps to ensure the person understands these rights.

Right of appeal (the right to appeal against being detained)?
None.

Right to an advocate?

No – there is no legal right to an *advocate* but the person may ask if one is available.

Right to be visited by and complain to the Care Quality Commission (CQC)?
Yes.

Discharge (how the Section ends)

1. The assessment for the Section 2 or 3 during the 72 hours decides that neither is needed.

2. The Section expires at the end of the 72 hours (this would be not considered good practice because detention should end as soon as it is no longer necessary)

Forms required

A magistrate's Section 135 (1) warrant.

Guidance (from the Act – Code of Practice)

Each Section 135 (1) warrant allows for forced entry to locked premises once only. The preferred *place of safety* is a hospital. A police station should only be used in exceptional circumstances. If possible, once entry is made, the doctor and AMHP should carry out an initial assessment to see whether any further assessments or treatment will be necessary – eg those required under Sections 2 and 3 of the Act.

Section 135 (2)

Purpose

The purpose of a Section 135(2) warrant is to provide police officers with a power of entry to private premises for the purposes of removing a patient who is liable to be taken or returned to hospital or any other place or into custody under the Act. The warrant must be granted by a magistrate. It enables a police officer to enter the premises, search for, and remove the patient so they can be taken to, or returned to, where they ought to be.

Legal criteria (these must be met to use the power of this Section)

There is reasonable cause to believe that a patient who is already subject to a section is to be found on the premises within the jurisdiction of the magistrate and admission to the premises has already been refused or a refusal of such admission is expected.

Duration of Section

Once the person is found, the original Section they were under (before they went AWOL) is reinstated and provides the authority to return them to hospital and resume their detention.

Professionals required to comply with and complete this Section

An authorised person from the hospital detaining or a police officer applies to a magistrate who issues a warrant.

A police officer then has authority to enter the premises.

Treatment (what are the treatment powers?)

Once found, a person comes under the *treatment* powers of the original Section under which they were detained.

Leave of absence?

Not applicable – the power is simply to search for an existing patient and return them.

Duties on staff

Staff must inform the person of their legal rights (both verbally and in writing) and take all practicable steps to ensure the person understands these rights.

Right of appeal (the right to appeal against being detained)?

None.

Right to an advocate?

No – there is no legal right to an *advocate* but the person may ask if one is available.

Right to be visited by and complain to the CQC?

Yes.

Discharge (how the Section ends)

The Section ends once the premises are entered and the person is found. The powers of the Section they were under at the time they went AWOL come into force.

Forms required

A magistrate's warrant.

Guidance (from the Act – Code of Practice)

The warrant must be used within one month of being issued. Informal attempts should be made to gain access first before forced entry under Section 135(2) is considered. It is good practice for the police officer to be accompanied by staff from the hospital or local authority is involved.

Section 136

Purpose

Police power to remove a person from a public place, who appears to have a *mental disorder*, for assessment in a *place of safety* (hospital or police station).

Legal criteria (these must be met to use the power of this Section)

> » A police officer finds, in a public place, a person who appears to be suffering from *mental disorder; and*
>
> » The person appears to be in immediate need of care of control; *and*
>
> » The police officer considers it necessary in the interests of that person or for the protection of others, to remove them to a *place of safety.*

Duration of Section

Up to 72 hours from the person's arrival at the *place of safety.*

Any further detention would require a new Section to be completed within the 72 hours – Section 2 or 3.

Professionals required to comply with and complete this Section

A police officer.

Treatment (what are the treatment powers?)

The person must consent to treatment or, if they lack capacity to consent, the Mental Capacity Act can be used to treat them in their best interests.

Leave of absence?

Not applicable – the power provides for short-term detention.

Duties on staff

Staff must inform the person of their legal rights (both verbally and in writing) and take all practicable steps to ensure the person understands these rights.

Right of appeal (the right to appeal against being detained)?

None.

Right to an advocate?

No – there is no legal right to an *advocate* but the person may ask if one is available.

Right to be visited by and complain to the CQC?

Yes.

Discharge (how the Section ends)

The person should be assessed by both a doctor *and* an Approved Mental Health Professional within the 72-hour period (see code of practice for when one person assesses). If the assessors do not feel any further detention is required the person can leave or admit themselves informally to hospital.

Forms required

Police form.

Guidance (from the Act – Code of Practice)

The preferred *place of safety* is a hospital and police stations should only be used in exceptional circumstances. A person can be transferred between different places of safety during the 72 hours. The *Code of Practice* has further information. The Royal College of Psychiatrists have standards for the use of Section 136.

Section 4

Purpose

The power to admit a person from the community to hospital and detain them there in an emergency.

Legal criteria (these must be met to use the power of this Section)

» It is of urgent necessity for the person to be admitted and detained under Section 2; *and*

» Compliance with the requirements of Section 2 (two doctors and an Approved Mental Health Professional) would involve unreasonable delay.

Duration of Section

» Up to 72 hours from when the person arrives at hospital.

» Any further detention would require a new Section (either Section 2 or 3) to be completed within a 72-hour period.

» Section 4 can be changed to a Section 2 by the addition of a second medical recommendation.

Professionals required to comply with and complete this Section

A doctor *and* an AMHP *(or* the *nearest relative).*

Treatment (what are the treatment powers?)

The person must either consent to treatment or, if they lack capacity to consent, the Mental Capacity Act may be used to treat their best interests.

Leave of absence?

Not applicable – the power provides for short-term detention.

Duties on staff

Staff must inform the person of their legal rights (both verbally and in writing) and take all practicable steps to ensure the person understands these rights.

Right of appeal (the right to appeal against being detained)?

None.

Right to an advocate?

No – there is no legal right to an *advocate* but the person may ask if one is available.

Right to be visited by and complain to the CQC?

Yes.

Discharge (how the Section ends)

1. The assessment for Section 2 or 3 concludes that neither is required.

2. The Section expires after 72 hours (this is not considered good practice because detention should end as soon as it is no longer necessary).

Forms required

» Form A9: Nearest relative *or*

» Form A10: Approved Mental Health Professional

» Form A11: Medical recommendation

» Form H3: Record of detention.

Guidance (from the Act – Code of Practice)

The person must be admitted to hospital within 24 hours of the earliest form being completed. Code of Practice: '*Section 4 should only be used in genuine emergency, where the patient's need for urgent assessment outweighs the desirability of waiting for a second doctor'* (paragraph 5.4).

Section 5 (2)

Purpose

To prevent an informal/voluntary patient leaving a ward in an emergency. This allows time to assess whether further detention (Section 2 or 3) is needed.

Legal criteria (these must be met to use the power of this section)

> » A person is a voluntary in-patient in hospital; *and*

> » It appears to a doctor or an *approved clinician* in charge of the person's *treatment* that an application ought to be made for a Section 2 or 3.

Duration of Section

Up to 72 hours – any further detention would require a new Section to be completed within a 72-hour period – Section 2 or 3.

Professionals required to comply with and complete this Section

A doctor *or* an approved clinician

Treatment (what are the treatment powers?)

The person must either consent to treatment or, if they lack capacity to consent, the Mental Capacity Act may be used to treat their best interests.

Leave of absence?

Not applicable – the power provides for short-term detention.

Duties on staff

Staff must inform the person of their legal rights (both verbally and in writing) and take all practicable steps to ensure the person understands these rights.

Right of appeal (the right to appeal against being detained)?

None.

Right to an advocate?

No – there is no legal right to an *advocate* but the person may ask if one is available.

Right to be visited by and complain to the CQC?

Yes.

Discharge (how the Section ends)

1. It is decided that further assessment for detention under Section 2 or 3 is not required.

2. The assessment for a Section 2 or 3 concludes that neither is required.

3. The Section expires at the end of the 72-hour period (this is not considered good practice because detention should end as soon as it is no longer necessary).

Forms required

Form H1: doctor or *approved clinician's* report on hospital in-patient.

Guidance (from the Act – Code of Practice)

The Code of Practice states: '*The power cannot be used for an out-patient attending a hospital's accident and emergency department or any other out-patients. Patients should not be admitted informally with the sole intention of then using the holding power*' (paragraph 12.7)

Section 5 (4)

Purpose

To prevent an informal/voluntary patient leaving a ward in an emergency. This allows time to complete a longer holding power.

Legal criteria (these must be met to use the power of this Section)

» A person is receiving treatment for *mental disorder* as an in-patient in hospital; *and*

» It appears to a nurse (of a prescribed level) that the disorder is of such a degree that is necessary for the person's health *or* safety *or* for the protection of others that they are immediately restrained from leaving hospital; *and*

» It is not practical to secure the immediate attendance of a person authorised to completed a Section 5(2).

Duration of Section

Up to six hours – any further detention would require a Section 5(2) to be completed within the six-hour period.

Professionals required to comply with and complete this Section

A registered nurse (registered with the Nursing and Midwifery Council as a Mental Health or Learning Disabilities Nurse).

Treatment (what are the treatment powers?)

The person must either consent to treatment or if they lack capacity to consent the Mental Capacity Act can be used to treat them in their best interests.

Leave of absence?

Not applicable – the power provides for short-term detention.

Duties on staff

Staff must inform the person of their legal rights (both verbally and in writing) and take all practicable steps to ensure the person understand these rights.

Right of appeal (the right to appeal against being detained)?

None.

Right to an advocate?

No – there is no legal right to an *advocate* but the person may ask if one is available.

Right to be visited by and complain to the CQC?

Yes.

Discharge (how the Section ends)

The Section is discharged when a doctor or *approved clinician* with authority to complete a Section 5(2) arrives within the six-hour period. This person will then decide whether a Section 5(2) is appropriate, if not, the Section ends. It is not good practice for the Section to run the full six hours and then expire; the doctor or *approved clinician* should arrive within that time.

Forms required

Form H2: Nurse's holding power.

Guidance (from the Act – Code of Practice)

The Code of Practice states: '*The decision to invoke the power is the personal decision of the nurse, who cannot be instructed to exercise the power by anyone else*' (Paragraph 12.25). '*The use of Section 5(4) is an emergency measure, and the doctor or approved clinician with the power to use section 5 (2) in respect of the patient should treat it as such and arrive as soon as possible*' (Paragraph 12.32).

Mental Health Act (1983) Sections – longer-term orders

Section 2

Purpose

To admit a person from the community to hospital or detain a patient wishing to leave hospital. It lasts for up to 28 days.

Legal criteria (these must be met to use the power of this Section)

> » A person is suffering from *mental disorder*; *and*
> » It is of a *nature* or *degree* which warrants their detention in hospital for assessment (or assessment followed by medical *treatment)* for at least a limited period; *and*
> » The person ought to be detained in the interests of their own health *or* safety *or* with the view to the protection of others.

Duration of Section

Up to 28 days.

Professionals required to comply with and complete this Section

Two doctors (one of whom must be Section 12 approved or an approved clinician) *and* an Approved Mental Health Professional (*or* the nearest relative).

Treatment (what are the treatment powers?)

Yes – *treatment* for mental disorder can be given whether the person consents, refuses or lacks capacity to give or refuse consent.

NB: The treatment rules are contained in Part 4 of the Act.

Leave of absence?

Yes – the *responsible clinician* can grant leave of absence.

Duties on staff

Staff must inform the person of their legal rights (both verbally and in writing) and take all practicable steps to ensure the person understands these rights.

Right of appeal (the right to appeal against being detained)?

Yes – a right of appeal to both the *Mental Health Tribunal* (the appeal must be made within 14 days of the Section 2 starting) and a right of appeal to the *hospital managers*.

Right to an advocate?

Yes.

Right to be visited by and complain to the CQC?

Yes.

Discharge (how the Section ends)

1. The responsible clinician at any time

2. Mental Health Tribunal

3. Hospital Managers' hearing

4. Nearest relative request

5. The Section expires at the end of the 28-day period (this is not considered good practice as detention should end as soon as it is no longer necessary).

Forms required

» Form A1: Nearest relative

» Form A2: Approved Mental Health Professional

» Form A3 or A4: medical recommendation

» Form H3: Record of detention.

Guidance (from the Act – Code of Practice)

Section 2 should be used if:

- » The full extent of the nature and degree of a patient's condition is unclear;
- » There is need to carry out an assessment to formulate a *treatment* plan or to reach a judgement about whether the patient will accept *treatment* on a voluntary basis following admission;
- » A new in-patient assessment is needed to re-formulate a *treatment* plan.

Section 3

Purpose

To admit a person from the community to hospital or to detain a patient wishing to leave hospital. It lasts for up to six months and can be renewed.

Legal criteria (these must be met to use the power of this section)

- » A person is suffering from *mental disorder; and*
- » It is of a *nature or degree* which makes it appropriate for them to receive medical *treatment* in hospital; *and*
- » It is necessary for the health *or* safety *or* with a view to the protection of others that they receive such *treatment* and *treatment* cannot be provided unless they are detained; *and*
- » Appropriate medical *treatment* is available for them.

Duration of Section

- » Up to six months initially – Section 3 can be renewed by the *responsible clinician.*
- » Up to six months for the first renewal and up to 12 months for each subsequent renewal.

Professionals required to comply with and complete this Section

Two doctors (one of whom must be Section 12 approved or an approved clinician) *and* an Approved Mental Health Professional (*or* the nearest relative).

Treatment (what are the treatment powers?)

Yes – *treatment* for mental disorder can be given whether the person consents, refuses or lacks capacity to give or refuse consent.

NB: The treatment rules are contained in Part 4 of the Act.

Leave of absence?

Yes – the *responsible clinician* can grant leave of absence.

Duties on staff

Staff must inform the person of their legal rights (both verbally and in writing) and take all practicable steps to ensure the person understands these rights.

Right of appeal (the right to appeal against being detained)?

Yes – a right of appeal to both the *Mental Health Tribunal* (the appeal must be made within 14 days of the Section 2 starting) and a right of appeal to the *hospital managers.*

Right to an advocate?

Yes.

Right to be visited by and complain to the CQC?

Yes.

Discharge (how the section ends)

1. The responsible clinician at any time

2. Mental Health Tribunals

3. Hospital Managers' hearing

4. Nearest relative request

5. Transfer to a Community Treatment Order

6. The Section expires (this is not considered good practice as detention should end as soon as it is no longer necessary).

Forms required

» Form A5: Nearest relative *or*

» Form A6: Approved Mental Health Professional

» Form A7 or A8: Medical recommendation

» Form H3: Record of detention.

Guidance (from the Act – Code of Practice)

The Code of Practice states: *'Section 3 should be used if:*

> » *the patient is already detained under Section 2; or*

> » *the nature and current degree of the patient's mental disorder, the essential elements of the treatment plan to be followed and the likelihood of the patient accepting treatment on a voluntary basis are already established'* (Para 4.27)

Section 37

Purpose

A person is found guilty of a crime and the court sentences them to hospital for *treatment.* It lasts for up to six months and can be renewed.

Legal criteria (these must be met to use the power of this Section)

> » A Magistrates' Court or a Crown Court convicts a person of an offence punishable with imprisonment and is of the opinion that Section 37 is the most suitable method of dealing with that person; *and*

> » They are suffering from *mental disorder* of a *nature or degree* which makes it appropriate for them to be detained in hospital for medical *treatment; and*

> » Appropriate medical *treatment* is available for them.

Duration of Section

Up to six months initially – Section 37 can be renewed by the *responsible clinician.*

Up to six months for the first renewal and up to 12 months for each subsequent renewal.

Professionals required to comply with and complete this Section

Two doctors (one of whom must be *Section 12 approved* or an *approved clinician) and* an order by a Magistrates' or Crown Court.

Treatment (what are the treatment powers?)

Yes – *treatment* for mental disorder can be given whether the person consents, refuses or lacks capacity to give or refuse consent.

NB: The treatment rules are contained in Part 4 of the Act.

Leave of absence?

Yes – the *responsible clinician* can grant leave of absence.

Duties on staff

Staff must inform the person of their legal rights (both verbally and in writing) and take all practicable steps to ensure the person understands these rights.

Right of appeal (the right to appeal against being detained)?

Yes – a right of appeal to both the *Mental Health Tribunal* (once in each period of detention) and a right of appeal to the *hospital managers* (at any time).

Right to an advocate?

Yes.

Right to be visited by and complain to the CQC?

Yes.

Discharge (how the section ends)

1. The responsible clinician at any time

2. Mental Health Tribunals

3. Hospital Managers' hearing

4. Nearest relative request

5. Transfer to a Community Treatment Order

6. The Section expires (this is not considered good practice as detention should end as soon as it is no longer necessary).

Forms required

The court issues a Section 37 Order.

Guidance (from the Act – Code of Practice)

If, at the time of sentencing, doctors are not satisfied that a hospital order is appropriate, they should consider a Section 38 interim order instead. This allows the hospital time to assess the patient to confirm whether a full hospital order is appropriate.

Courts can also make a Section 37 as a guardianship order in the community instead.

Mental Health Act (1983) – Community Treatment Order (CTO)

Purpose

The power for a hospital to discharge a detained patient into the community under a CTO. They become subject to conditions enforceable by the power to recall the person back to hospital.

In the event of recall back to hospital and revocation (ending) of the CTO, the original hospital section they were discharged from begins again.

Legal criteria (these must be met to use the power of this section)

» A patient is detained under either Section 3, 37, 45A, 47, 48; *and*

» Has a *mental disorder* of a *nature* or *degree* which makes it appropriate for them to receive medical *treatment*; *and*

» It is necessary for their health *or* safety *or* for the protection of others that they should receive treatment; *and*

» Subject to them being liable to be recalled such *treatment* can be provided without them continuing to be detained in hospital; *and*

» It is necessary that the *responsible clinician* should be able to exercise the power to recall the person to hospital; *and*

» Appropriate medical *treatment* is available for them.

Duration of Section

Up to six months initially – It can be renewed by the *responsible clinician.*
Up to six months for the first renewal and up to 12 months for each subsequent renewal.

Professionals required to comply with and complete this Section

The responsible clinician *and* an Approved Mental Health Professional.

Treatment (what are the treatment powers?)

If they have capacity, the person must consent to treatment. If they lack capacity to consent, treatment can be given under the powers of the CTO. In all cases (including overriding a valid refusal of consent) *treatment* can be given if they are recalled back to hospital.

Leave of absence?

Not applicable as the person is not detained in hospital

Duties on staff

Staff must inform the person their legal rights (both verbally and in writing) and take all practicable steps to ensure the person understands these rights.

Right of appeal (the right to appeal against being detained)?

Yes – a right of appeal to both the *Mental Health Tribunal* (once during each period of CTO) and a right of appeal to the *Hospital Managers* at any time.

Right to an advocate?

Yes.

Right to be visited by and complain to the CQC?

Yes.

Discharge (how the section ends)

1. The responsible clinician at any time
2. The person is recalled and then the CTO is revoked (they are under their original detention section)
3. Mental Health Tribunal
4. Hospital Managers' hearing
5. Nearest relative's request
6. The CTO expires (this is not considered good practice as the CTO should end as soon as it is no longer required).

Forms required

Form CTO1.

Guidance (from the Act – Code of Practice)

A patient with history of non-compliance with treatment plans or medication while in the community, resulting in relapse, may justify the use of a CTO as opposed to discharge.

The conditions should restrict the patient's liberty as little as possible while still achieving their purpose.

Mental Health Act (1983) – Guardianship

Purpose

The power for a guardian (usually someone in the local authority) to manage a person's care in the community (including deciding where they should live, whether they should attend appointments, education and training).

Guardianship does not provide the power to detain.

Legal criteria (these must be met to use the power of this section)

- » A person is 16+ years old; *and*
- » Has a *mental disorder*; and
- » The *mental disorder* is not of a *nature* or *degree* to warrant the need for guardianship; *and*
- » It is necessary in the interests of the welfare of the person **or** for the protection of others that guardianship is used.

Duration of Section

Up to six months initially – it can be renewed (usually by the *responsible clinician).*
Up to six months for the first renewal and up to 12 months for each subsequent renewal.

Professionals required to comply with and complete this Section

Two doctors (one of whom must be Section 12 approved or an approved clinician) *and* an Approved Mental Health Professional (or nearest relative).

Treatment (what are the treatment powers?)

Guardianship gives no authority to treat. The person must consent to treatment or, if they lack capacity, treatment may be provided under the Mental Capacity Act in their best interests.

Leave of absence?

Not applicable as the person is not detained in hospital.

Duties on staff

Staff must inform the person of their legal rights (both verbally and in writing) and take all practicable steps to ensure the person understands these rights.

Right of appeal (the right to appeal against being detained)?

Yes – a right of appeal to both the Mental Health Tribunal (once during each period of the guardianship) and a right of appeal to the local authority.

Right to an advocate?

Yes.

Right to be visited by and complain to the CQC?

Yes.

Discharge (how the section ends)

1. The responsible clinician authorised by local authority

2. The responsible local authority

3. Mental Health Tribunal

4. Nearest relative

5. Transfer of hospital and then detention under Section 3

6. The guardianship order expires (this is not considered good practice as detention should end as soon as it is no longer necessary).

Forms required

- »   Form G1: nearest relative *or*

- »   Form G2: Approved Mental Health Professional

- »   Form G3 or G4: medical recommendation

- »   Form G5: record of acceptance.

Guidance (from the Act – Code of Practice)

If a person consistently refuses the guardian's authority to make decisions, consideration should be given to an alternative guardian.

A person subject to guardianship can be admitted to hospital informally for their mental health.

Detention does not automatically become necessary just because they have been subject to guardianship.

Terminology

Advocate (IMHA)

IMHA stands for Independent Health Advocate. This is a professional advocate (not a lawyer) whose role is to help and support people detained under the Act. The majority of detained patients have a legal right to see one (free of charge) and the hospital detaining the patient has a duty to inform the person of this right. Even if a person does not have a right to an IMHA under their Section they can still ask if an advocate is available to help them.

Approved Clinician (AC)

A doctor, nurse or psychologist, social worker or occupational therapist who has undertaken specific training in connection with the Act for the purpose of this role. An approved clinician has a number of powers and duties under the Act, including to detain under Section 5(2).

Approved Mental Health Professional – (AMHP)

A Social Worker, nurse, psychologist or occupational therapist who has undertaken specific training in connection with the Act for the purpose of this role.

An AMHP has a number of powers and duties which include:

> » Making assessments for admission under Sections 2, 3 and 4;

> » Assigning and consulting nearest relatives for Sections 2 and 3;

> » Confirming that Community Treatment Orders should be made.

Care Quality Commission (CQC)

The independent regulatory body for the NHS and other care providers. All detained patients have a right to be visited by and complain to the Care Quality Commission.

Contact details:

Phone number: 03000 616 161

Website: www.cqc.org.uk

Code of Practice

The Act has a statutory Code of Practice which gives advice on best practice when using legislation. All staff have a duty in law to have 'regard to' the Code of Practice. The most recent copy of the Code of Practice can be found on the Department of Health website.

Hospital Managers

An independent group of people with relevant experience (not managers from the hospital itself) can hear appeals from people detained under some sections. A hospital managers' hearing consists of three such people who meet the patient and those involved in their care and decide whether to discharge the patient from their detention. Patients who appeal have a right to ask for a solicitor to help them. This can be free of charge but patients must speak to the solicitor to confirm this.

Mental Disorder

Defined in the Act as any 'disorder or disability of the mind'. Examples include:

- » Depression
- » Bipolar disorder
- » Schizophrenia
- » Anxiety
- » Phobic disorders
- » Obsessive compulsive disorders
- » Post-traumatic stress
- » Dementia
- » Delirium
- » Personality and behavioural changes due to brain injury
- » Personality disorders
- » Eating disorders
- » Autistic spectrum disorders

NB: If a person has learning difficulties and detention under Section 3, 37, Guardianship or a Community Treatment Order is being considered, the learning difficulties MUST be 'associated with abnormally aggressive or seriously irresponsible conduct' (this also applies to the court/prison Sections 35, 36, 38, 45A, 47 and 48 – these are not detailed through the guide).

Mental Health Tribunal

An independent tribunal that can discharge a detained patient's Section. The tribunal consists of three people who meet the patient and those involved in their care to decide whether to discharge. Patients who appeal have a right to ask a solicitor to help them and this is free of charge.

Contact details:

Phone number: 0845 2232 022

Website: www.mhrt.org.uk

Nature or degree

For some sections, a person's mental disorder must be of a 'nature or degree' to warrant detention. Both do not need to be present to warrant detention. The Code of Practice explains that: *'Nature refers to particular mental disorder from which the patient is suffering, its chronicity, its prognosis and the patient's previous response to receiving treatment for the disorder. Degree refers to the current manifestation of the patient's disorder.'*

Nearest relative

People detained under the longer-term sections of the Act are allocated a nearest relative who has certain powers. An Approved Mental Health Professional will decide who to appoint as nearest relative based on the hierarchy and the rules contained within the Act. If a person is not happy with the choice that the nearest relative made, they can contest this in court. An advocate or an Approved Mental Health Professional should be able to provide help in relation to this.

Place of Safety

Is defined as a hospital, police station, social services residential unit, care home [for mental disordered persons] or any other suitable place the occupier of which is willing to temporarily receive the patient.

Responsible Clinician (RC)

Detained patients may have had several approved clinicians involved in their care but only one of them will be the responsible clinician. Generally this will be the doctor in charge of a person's care (however, it could be a nurse, psychologist, social worker, or occupational therapist qualified to act as an approved clinician). A responsible clinician has authority under the Act to make certain decisions regarding detained patients – for example, give them leave or absence or to discharge them.

Section 12 approved

A doctor who has undertaken training on the Act and is approved to carry out medical assessments in order to detain people.

Treatment

The power to treat people with or without consent is contained in the Act for longer detention sections. Medical treatment for mental disorder is defined by the Act (Section 145) and includes nursing care, psychological intervention and specialist mental health rehabilitation and care. This means a range of treatments including medication, care to alleviate symptoms of the disorder, nursing care, monitoring blood where this is part of taking certain medication, diagnostic tests for mental disorder and the care provided while a patient is in seclusion are covered. General medical treatment may also be given if it can be shown to be treating a symptom directly resulting from the patient's mental disorder or integral to it. For example, the use of nasal-gastric tube feeding in the case of a patient with anorexia nervosa.

Appendix 3: A simple guide to terminology in Safeguarding Adults

Term	Replaces (as applicable)	Comment
Safeguarding Concern	Alert	Levels no longer apply. Nature of concern, risk and outcome(s) the adult wants to achieve informs what is the most appropriate and proportionate response to the concern, eg causing an enquiry to be made by another organisation/agency.
Three Tests in the Care Act (2014)	N/A	Three key tests in relation to adults covered by the safeguarding procedures. The safeguarding duties apply to an adult who: • has needs for care and support (whether or not the local authority is meeting any of those needs); and • is experiencing, or is at risk of, abuse or neglect; and • as a result of those care and support needs is unable to protect themselves from the risk or experience of abuse or neglect. Once the local authority has reasonable cause to believe an adult meets this test its Section 42 Duty is triggered. The local authority may still decide to undertaken an Enquiry where the three tests in the Care Act are not met. NB: Carers are also covered by the procedures where they meet the three tests set out above.
Safeguarding Enquiry	Investigation	An 'Enquiry' is any first action taken in response to a Safeguarding Concern to establish whether the local authority's Section 42 duty has been triggered, ie the three tests in the Care Act have been met. There is a move away from investigations (except by the Police and where disciplinary investigations are undertaken by employers).
Section 42 (S.42) Enquiry	Investigation	The local authority must make or cause other agencies/organisations to make Enquiries when its Section 42 duty is triggered, ie when it has reasonable cause to believe that the three tests in the Care Act have been met.
Initial Actions (Enquiries)	N/A	Any first responses made under the local authority's Section 42 Duty to make Enquiries/cause enquiries to be made. As a means of embedding Making Safeguarding Personal (MSP) into the Enquiry a conversation with the adult should always be the first response (or one of the first responses if they have not already been spoken with).

Term	Replaces (as applicable)	Comment
Conclusion of an Enquiry	N/A	The local authority's Section 42 duty of enquiry continues until it has decided what action is necessary to protect the adult, and by whom, and has ensured that this action has been taken.
Further Actions (Enquiries)	N/A	If the issue cannot be resolved through the actions taken in the initial response to the Safeguarding Concern the local authority's duty under Section 42 continues until it decides what action is necessary to protect the adult, and by whom, and ensures itself that this action has been taken.
Enquiry Manager	Investigation Manager	A suitably trained and experienced practitioner employed by the local authority with responsibility for decision-making in relation Section 42 Enquiries.
Enquirer	Investigating Officer	A suitably trained and skilled practitioner undertaking an Enquiry or aspects of an Enquiry.
Safeguarding Adults Review (SAR)	Serious Case Review	Safeguarding Adults Boards must arrange a SAR when an adult in its area dies as a result of, or has experienced, serious abuse or neglect (known or suspected) and there is concern that partner agencies could have worked more effectively together. The aim of the SAR is to identify and implement learning from this.
The person(s)/ service thought to be the cause of risk	Person/Service alleged to be responsible	A person, organisation/service who may have some relationship to the cause of risk or issue of concern for the adult.
Types of abuse	Categories of abuse	These are types of abuse identified in the Care Act guidance. In addition to the existing types of abuse, domestic violence, modern slavery and self-neglect are now included.
Organisational abuse	Institutional abuse	Includes neglect and poor practice within an institution or specific care setting, eg in a hospital or care home or in relation to care provided in a person's own home. This may range from 'one-off' incidents to ongoing ill-treatment. It can be through neglect or poor professional practice as a result of the structure, policies, processes and practices within an organisation.
Modern Slavery	N/A	Includes slavery, human trafficking, forced labour, and domestic servitude, including inhumane and abusive treatment.
Domestic Abuse	N/A	NB: Safeguarding Adults procedures are concerned with people aged 18 and over. Domestic Violence includes young people aged 16 years and over; however, young people are covered by Child Protection procedures.

Term	Replaces (as applicable)	Comment
Self-neglect	N/A	In brief: the inability or unwillingness to undertake or complete essential personal or environmental health and safety tasks (NB: Refer to more comprehensive definition of this complex and multi-faceted issue)
Planning Meeting Outcome Meeting	Strategy Meeting Case Conference	Safeguarding Adults work and a 'Making Safeguarding Personal' (MSP) approach starts from the point that the adult/their representative will always be included in any discussion or meeting that relates to them.
Adult	Adult at risk	A person who meets the three key tests set out in the Care Act.
Harm		A negative or detrimental impact on an adult's emotional, physical or mental well-being.
Making Safeguarding Personal (MSP)		'Making Safeguarding Personal' means person-led and outcomes focused. It engages the person in a conversation about how best to respond to their safeguarding situation in a way that enhances their involvement, choice and control as well as improving quality of life, well-being and safety.
Safeguarding Plan		Actions/arrangements agreed with the adult to support them in maintaining their safety. These should be incorporated into the adult's support/care plan where they have one. It should include clear information regarding roles and responsibilities of all those involved and the arrangements for monitoring and reviewing the effectiveness of this plan.
		Where there are actions that relate to the local authority and/or other agencies, rather than the individual adult, these should also be recorded.
		While the local authority's Section 42 duty will be discharged once it has determined that the adult has been protected and/or the actions required have been taken, it must ensure that any actions taken as a result of this process are effectively monitored and reviewed.
		This may include actions for agencies and organisations where the adult does not wish to have a Safeguarding Plan in place.
Agencies responsible for commissioning/ commissioners		The term 'commissioning' or 'commissioners' refers to any agency, service or team with a responsibility for commissioning care and support service, including social care, health, housing etc. It includes any commissioning and quality assurance functions, and teams with this function.

Term	Replaces (as applicable)	Comment
Deprivation of Liberty Safeguards (DOLS)		The Mental Capacity Act Deprivation of Liberty Safeguards (DOLS) were created as an amendment to the Mental Capacity Act 2005 (introduced by the Mental Health Act 2007) to provide a legal process to authorise the deprivation of liberty of a person in a hospital or care home who lacks Capacity to consent.
Court of Protection		The specialist Court for all issues relating to people who lack capacity to make specific decisions. The Court of Protection was established under Section 45 of the Mental Capacity Act 2005 (MCA).
Care Quality Commission (CQC)		The Care Quality Commission (CQC) is the independent regulator of health and social care in England. They regulate care provided by the NHS, local authorities, private companies and voluntary organisations. They aim to make sure better care is provided for everyone – in hospitals, care homes and people's own homes. They also seek to protect the interests of people whose rights are restricted under the Mental Health Act.

Index

Printed in the United States
by Baker & Taylor Publisher Services